I0078637

AUTHENTIC
Beauty

W

WELLSPRINGS
BOOKS

Paducah, Kentucky

W

WELLSPRINGS

BOOKS

Authentic Beauty: Reclaiming Health While Reflecting the Image of God by Evelyn M. Jones, MD

Copyright © 2024 Evelyn M. Jones

Published in 2024 by Wellsprings Books
2721 West Park Dr., Paducah, Kentucky 42001
https://drevelynjones.com

All rights reserved. No part of the contents of this book may be reproduced by any means without the written permission of the publisher.

Medical disclaimer: Although the publisher and the author have made every effort to ensure that the information in this book was correct at press time and while this publication is designed to provide accurate information in regard to the subject matter covered, the publisher and the author assume no responsibility for errors, inaccuracies, omissions, or any other inconsistencies herein and hereby disclaim any liability to any party for any loss, damage, or disruption caused by errors or omissions, whether such errors or omissions result from negligence, accident, or any other cause. This publication is meant as a source of valuable information for the reader, however it is not meant as a substitute for direct expert assistance. If such level of assistance is required, the services of a competent professional should be sought.

Scripture quotations taken from the (NASB®) New American Standard Bible®, Copyright © 1960, 1971, 1977, 1995, 2020 by The Lockman Foundation. Used by permission. All rights reserved. lockman.org. This is the predominant version used. Where marked NIV, Scripture is taken from THE HOLY BIBLE, NEW INTERNATIONAL VERSION®, NIV® Copyright © 1973, 1978, 1984, 2011 by Biblica, Inc.® Used by permission. All rights reserved worldwide. Scripture quotations are from The ESV® Bible (The Holy Bible, English Standard Version®), © 2001 by Crossway, a publishing ministry of Good News Publishers. Used by permission. All rights reserved. Scripture quotations marked (NLT) are taken from the Holy Bible, New Living Translation, copyright ©1996, 2004, 2015 by Tyndale House Foundation. Used by permission of Tyndale House Publishers, Carol Stream, Illinois 60188. All rights reserved. Scripture quotations marks NRSV are from New Revised Standard Version Bible, copyright © 1989 National Council of the Churches of Christ in the United States of America. Used by permission. All rights reserved worldwide. Scripture quotations taken from the Amplified® Bible (AMP), Copyright © 2015 by The Lockman Foundation. Used by permission. lockman.org. Scripture taken from the New King James Version®. Copyright © 1982 by Thomas Nelson. Used by permission. All rights reserved.

ISBN: 979-8-9903801-0-3

Publishing and design services: MelindaMartin.me
Editors: Kristin Demery and Gail Fallen
Cover stock art: https://www.shutterstock.com/g/LeandroLugones

AUTHENTIC
Beauty

RECLAIMING HEALTH
While Reflecting *the* IMAGE *of* GOD

Evelyn M. Jones, MD
BOARD CERTIFIED DERMATOLOGIST

(W)

WELLSPRINGS
BOOKS

Paducah, Kentucky

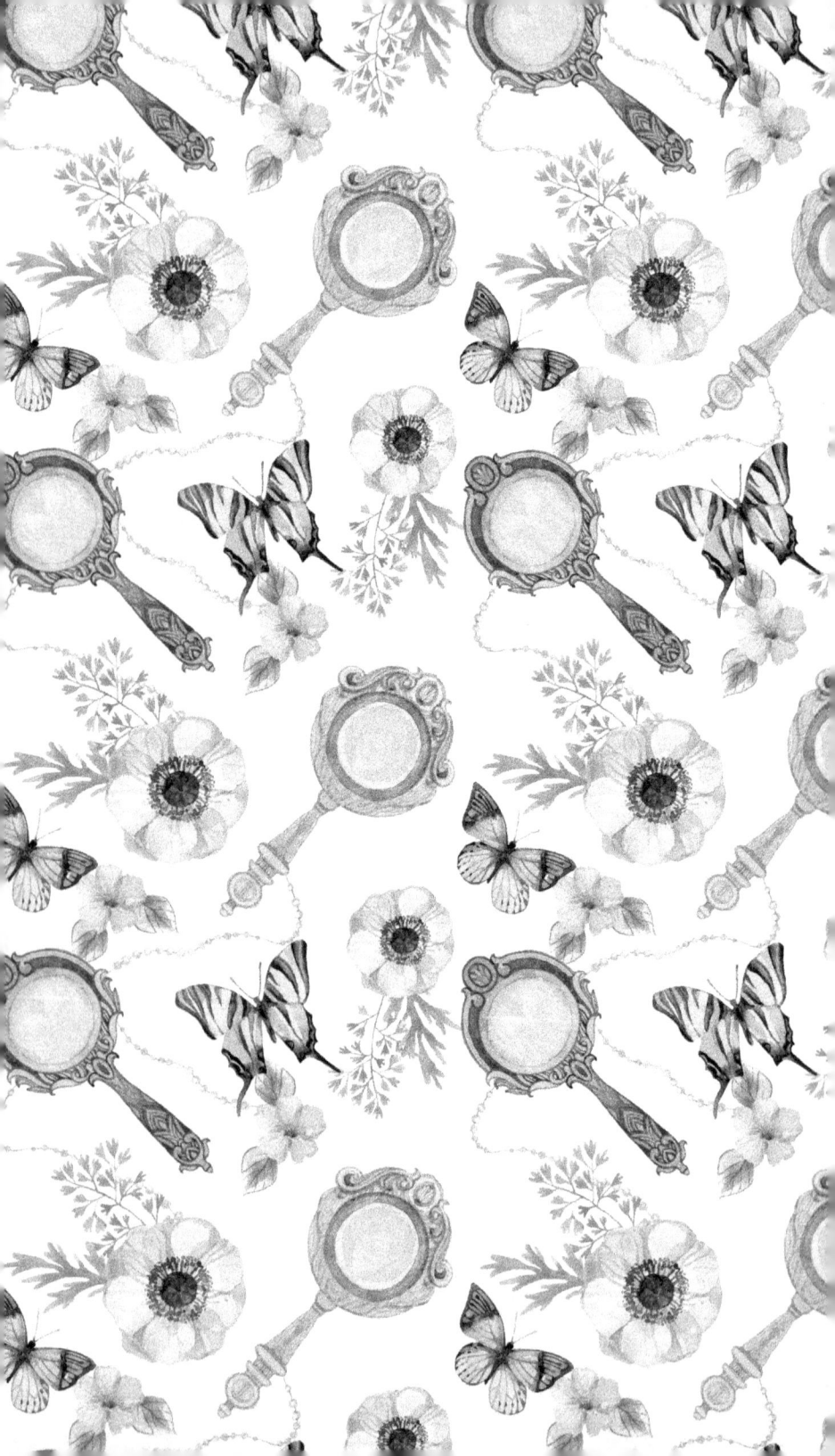

DEDICATION

To the strong, authentically beautiful women in my family: My grandmothers who loved me so well, Evelyn Audelle Biggs and Katharine Montgomery. To my strong, determined, visionary mother, Gerry Biggs Montgomery, who encouraged me to believe in myself. To my dear, brilliant and beautiful daughter, Rebecca Evelyn Antwi who inspires me to be truly and unapologetically authentic. To my lovely, intelligent and compassionate daughter-in-love, Claire Elizabeth Jones, who invites me into her heart and mind openly and authentically.

To the compassionate, intelligent, supportive men in my life, who have loved me well: To my grandfathers, James Biggs who instilled deep integrity and work ethic, and Albert Montgomery, who taught me to love life and embrace each day with a little mischief and fun. To my father, who loved me in his special way and encouraged me to bring all of me to every person I met. My husband, Shawn Jones, who has seen the best of me and the worst of me and yet still loves, encourages and supports me in every way. I adore you honey. To my sons, Shawn Curtis and Caleb, who embrace their unique selves and share themselves with me at every opportunity. To my son-in-love, Christian Antwi, who has opened my mind and heart to truly see all people and have a desire to love them, know them and accept them.

To God, who has continually put people in my path to point me to You, Your Word, Your son Jesus and the hope of Heaven, my true home.

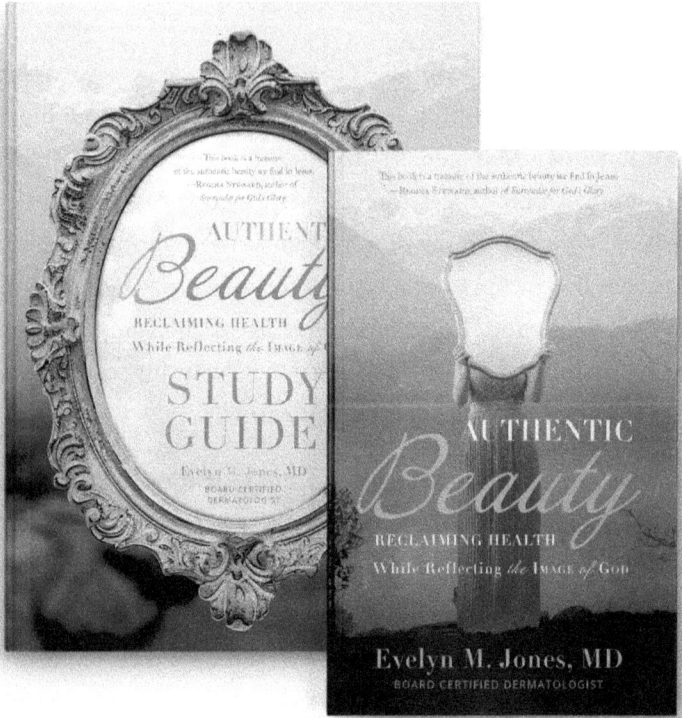

The *Authentic Beauty Study Guide*
is available on Amazon.

Live Authentically.
Grow Deeply. Reflect His Beauty.

*T*HE *AUTHENTIC BEAUTY STUDY GUIDE* IS DESIGNED TO help you not only read but also live out the truths found in *Authentic Beauty*. With reflection questions, scripture references, prayer journaling prompts, and practical "SNAP" practices (Seek Him, Nourish Self, Armor of God, Prayer), this workbook will guide you to embrace your God-given worth from the inside out.

Whether used in personal devotion or small group study, this companion will help you:

- Anchor your identity in Christ, not culture.

- Make daily choices that honor God with your body, mind, and soul.

- Cultivate healthy choices of food, movement, relationships, and words.

- Embrace stewardship, serving and freedom through Christ's transforming work.

- Record prayers, insights, and steps of growth as you journey toward lasting beauty and vitality.

Dr. Evelyn M. Jones invites you to take this next step—moving from inspiration to transformation. With space for reflection, room for prayer, and encouragement for action, the *Authentic Beauty Study Guide* will equip you to live courageously, love deeply, and walk in the fullness of God's design.

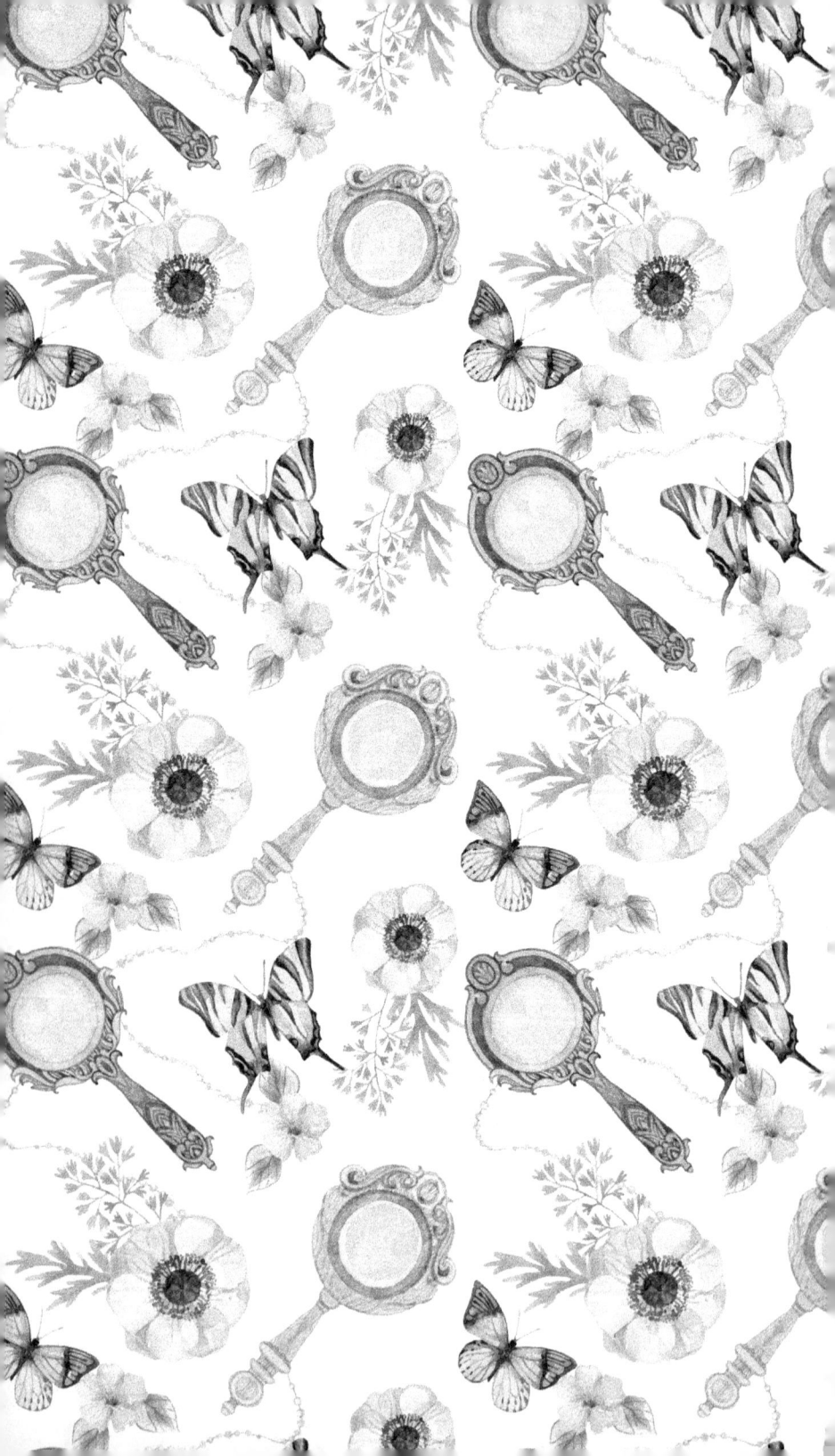

CONTENTS

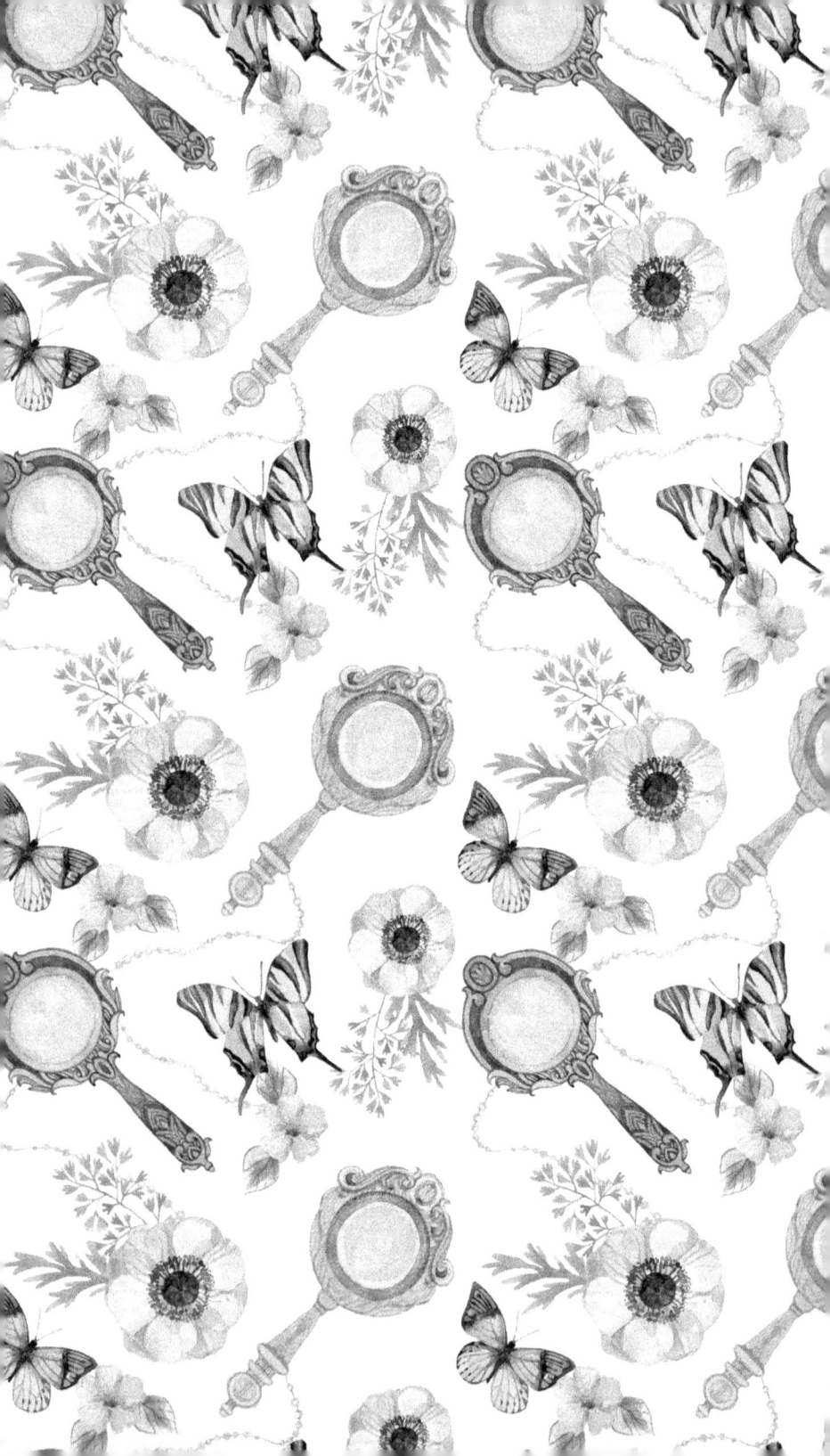

Introduction

*W*E WERE ON VACATION AT THE "HAPPIEST PLACE ON Earth" when I passed out in the bathroom. This moment was the beginning of the long journey toward regaining my health. Instead of relying on the few hours of biochemistry dedicated to nutrition in medical school, I had to learn about nutrition from a very personal vantage point. I had to figure out how to be healthy rather than just look healthy.

From the outside, I was doing well. I was a practicing dermatologist who owned my own practice and worked three to four days a week, doing some administrative work on other days. I was married to a man I love dearly and had three amazing children. I cooked meals most nights. I was a room mother and attended every possible activity I could at school. We were in church several times a week. We had breakfast every morning before sending the kids off to school. We exercised and ate fairly well.

Despite all this, I was struggling. For years, I had hidden the pain I felt. I'd struggled to overcome the abuse I experienced as a toddler and teenager. I'd endured the heartaches of loneliness in marriage and the lack of trust in relationships. I'd experienced the ups and downs of financial business challenges as the sole owner of my own medical practice and retail skincare company. I spent years on the roller coaster battle of a chronic autoimmune disease. I'd felt the heartache of caring for a parent at the end of their life and the grief of a loved one's slow slide into dementia.

And though I've always been someone with a "can do" mentality, on the day I passed out, I realized that I couldn't muscle my way through life anymore. The truth, the hurt, and the stress of my wounding were destroying me from the inside out.

From that day on, the stress I faced required me to deepen my understanding of foods to promote health and fight off chronic disease; to find a way to strengthen myself intentionally, not just when I had time; to explore meditation, mindfulness, and sleep etiquette; and to live out letting go and letting God.

After years of listening to the stories of those around me, I know I'm not alone. I have walked alongside countless women as patients or attendees of my seminars and heard their own painful stories of hidden sorrow.

Over time, I've realized that we all want the same things. We all want to feel beautiful; to be seen, known, and heard; to trust we are making a difference; to rise above the fray of the comparison cycle and our inner critic; and to decipher the best choices to make for ourselves and our loved ones when it comes to our spiritual, physical, and emotional well-being.

I cannot pretend to know your journey and story that has led you to a place where you do not feel beautiful or see your authentic beauty. I also do not know the specific health challenges and obstacles you face in making lifestyle choices to promote your optimum health. However, I do know my journey and struggle for acceptance. And I also understand the beautiful gift of forgiveness, acceptance, surrender, and trust as a choice despite the circumstances.

As you open this book to read, I encourage you to embrace all the aspects of your authentically beautiful self. I desire to sit with you, lean in, and listen to you describe your personality's facets as you rest in knowing your incredible value and worth. My prayer is that this will serve as a guide to truly believing and owning your authentic beauty and a resource for daily choices that help steward your health to gain true vitality.

Authentic Beauty will take us on an inward journey toward understanding the "why" behind the lifestyle choices that we make for our mind, body, and soul. Next, we'll begin to reclaim our authentic beauty and unapologetically drop the cultural pressures around nutrition, exercise, social media, conversations, thoughts, intellectual pursuits, makeup, and skin care. The last few chapters will focus on staying the course, extending and receiving grace, and choosing to live abundantly with health, hope, and vitality. The Lord calls us in Matthew 22:37–39 to love Him with all our heart, soul, strength, and mind and to love our neighbor as we love ourselves. We are free to love Him, to love ourselves, and to love others. That is authentic beauty. Caring for your health and beauty isn't a matter of vanity; it's a God-given priority.

My hope and prayer in writing this book is to help you recognize your true value in God, gain peace in knowing He loves you unconditionally, and allow you to soar in this life. My goal is to help you gain the confidence you need to grow beyond comparisons and to grab on to the abundant life God has promised.

Each chapter will close with a SNAP summary: **S**eek Him, **N**ourish Self, **A**rmor of God, and **P**rayer. These summaries will help you synthesize the information you've learned, providing clarity amid the day's chaos. Living with authentic beauty and health is not difficult, but it must be intentional. You'll find this quick summary at the end of each chapter.

Let us learn from one another, encourage one another, and begin afresh each new day with the Lord's promises.

"Hear, O Lord, and be gracious to me; O Lord, be my helper. Thou hast turned for me my mourning into dancing: Thou hast loosed my sackcloth, and girded me with gladness; That my soul may sing praise to Thee, and not be silent. O Lord my God, I will give thanks to Thee forever" (Ps. 30:10–12 KJV).

May we believe in His love and live from that place. Let's begin, beloved.

CHAPTER 1

Mirror, Mirror, on the Wall

"*Y*ou are beautiful!" The life coach's words were confident, her gaze unwavering as I shifted uncomfortably in my chair. We'd met at a small restaurant in my hometown of Paducah, Kentucky, to continue our work together. My business was at a crossroads, and I sought her help to understand better the complex situation and my path moving forward. I hadn't realized how vulnerable it would feel to delve deep into my strengths, weaknesses, and motivations.

As I rolled my eyes and looked away, she reiterated her words: "I would love for you to see the beauty that I see in you. I would love for you to accept and know you are beautiful."

Though I tried to brush off her words, they took hold in the tender places in my heart. The emotional and physical wounding of my past had led me to a place where I did not see my beauty and did not feel beautiful. So how could someone else see it in me?

What is beauty? Is it something someone sees from the outside—our size, hair, or clothing? Is it revealed by the words we speak from the heart that allow our authentic beauty to radiate outward? Is it the divine spark deep within us that shines through with love, joy, confidence, and hope? The answers to these questions are powerful, and our journey will take us to a place where we desire and have permission to embrace the authentic, beautiful self that God made. This journey will help us steward our lives in a way that honors God in our healthy choices, deepens our hope in the life ahead, and prepares us to live a life of beautiful vitality.

As a dermatologist, my days over the last thirty years have been filled with patients of all ages struggling with skin problems. From an outside perspective, this may seem like a superficial profession based on external beauty. However, each day is diverse and filled with amazing people who desire their skin to look and feel different or better.

Over the years, I've connected with all kinds of people:

- The teenager with bad acne who wouldn't look me in the eye, tried to cover their face with their hair, and possessed a subdued spirit who—once treated and sporting a new hairstyle—was animated, alive, and confident.

- The woman who experienced the itching and misery of full-body hives who was not at all self-conscious about disrobing in the hope of finding relief.

- The five-year-old boy who had horribly thick, scaly plaques of eczema covering his face and body. His guidance counselor shared that he was being made fun of at school, avoided, and ostracized by the other children. Yet once his skin cleared, he jumped into my arms at our follow-up appointment and pulled out $1.30 from his pocket—his lunch money—that he had saved to give as a thank you. Though I declined his sweet gratuity, I welcomed his hug.

Dermatology is more than skin deep—just like authentic beauty. Society's standards for beauty and self-worth are a moving target that focuses on appearance, achievement, approval, and affluence. But when we learn to see ourselves as God sees us, our self-worth and ability to recognize our authentic beauty change dramatically. As Christians, we can define ourselves by God's unconditional love for us, which never changes. God defines authentic beauty.

Jesus notices you, sees you, and says you matter to Him. As Luke 12:6–7 (NASB 1995) reminds us, "Are not five sparrows sold for two cents? And yet not one of them is forgotten before God. Indeed the very hairs of your head are all numbered, do not fear; you are of more value than many sparrows."

When we begin making choices that honor God and ourselves, we are free to look in the mirror and love ourselves for who He has made us to be. This is the true transformation that Paul alludes to in 2 Corinthians 3:18, "But we all, with unveiled face, beholding as in a mirror the glory of the Lord, are being transformed into the same image from glory to glory, just as from the Lord, the Spirit." Let us pause momentarily, look in the mirror, gaze at ourselves the way He does—with "shouts of joy" (Zeph. 3:17)—and then go about our day with health, hope, and vitality.

Choosing to Look in the Mirror

I felt more nervous than usual for a speaking engagement. This conference for women was a weekend event, and I was only scheduled to speak for one hour, so the commitment was less than usual for me. I had planned to be more direct in this talk as I listened to what was stirring inside me.

But my nerves were telling me that skirting along the edge would not be well-received, and maybe I should rethink and pull back a little. *Would I offend anyone? Would these women hear my heart in the delivery of the challenges I would make to them and myself?*

As the applause that followed my introduction broke out, I made my way to the podium. I am a planner by nature; changing my talk on a whim just does not happen. But after a few introductory words of gratitude, I began to speak. I had prayed about this message, and I trusted God to be faithful to hear my prayer. I felt as though the words I offered were truly His.

Midway through the talk, I asked the ladies in the room to pick up the small handheld mirror at their table, look into it, and name three things they loved about themselves. I began this exercise with an example of my own:

- *I love my green eyes because they remind me of my mother's eyes and my grandmother's eyes. These two women had been examples of powerful, diligent, intelligent women with a heart of compassion.*

- *I love my smile as I use it to spread pockets of sunshine to the people I meet.*

- *I love my hands because they allow me to do surgery on my patients and remind me of my father teaching me to suture. He was a general surgeon who has since passed away.*

It was not easy to mention these positive traits without instantly thinking of several negative ones, but that was the point.

I reminded the women that their words could be nothing negative, only positive. The room was very quiet at first. Then, a few whispers gained momentum and became scattered talk. Laughter broke out, and then, finally, tears. Why is it so challenging to love ourselves and recognize the authentic beauty we embody? There is so much to love about ourselves. Yet we are our own worst critics.

Investigating Our Barriers to Health

One of the most memorable parts of a medical mission trip to Honduras that my family and I took together was a recurring scenario each time I stopped and pulled my camera out of my pocket. After I took the photo, they would sidle up close to me or tug on my arm, wanting desperately to see the image. As soon as they saw it and spotted themselves in the picture—full disclosure, we all look at ourselves first when we see a picture—they would smile. They would beam with joy. I realized that they do not have mirrors or cameras. They likely do not know what they look like. Yet when they saw themselves, they experienced full-on joy. They loved themselves. They loved seeing their image reflected in the photograph. Do you and I feel this way? In a culture where we have plenty of mirrors, cameras, and selfies, do we love what we see?

The contrast between that joyful experience on the mountain and the day-to-day reality of my dermatology practice—where women constantly speak negative messages about themselves—was quite stark.

My days take me into the world of skin. Dermatology is a very external-focused profession. The skin is the body's largest organ, covers our entire being, and reflects what is happening inside us. I teach my patients that truly healthy skin is beautiful skin. Though beauty standards often focus on all the wrong things—weight, size, skin color, hair, or abilities—a healthy relationship with our Creator allows our authentic beauty to shine. Our beauty, external and internal, is all from Him. We can choose a different focus than our culture and reframe the conversation around beauty to combat the erosion of self-worth. We are worthy, beautiful, and precious to the core. Yet rejection can paralyze us from living with confidence.

Why is there such a gap between the joy I witnessed in Honduras and the quiet desperation I hear daily in the US? Is it because our perspective influences our thoughts? After all, when we first begin to rustle around in our beds and flutter open our eyes, we choose the perspective we will bring to the day ahead. We decide how we will think about our circumstances. We are the ones who walk into our bathroom, look in the mirror, and make judgments about ourselves. Though the person reflected at us remains fairly consistent, our perception is influenced by a waterfall of feelings, hurts, words, and wounding from other people as well as our inner critic.

From the time I was a little girl, I remember the wounds from others that made me feel small and unworthy. I remember my sadness, red cheeks, and broken heart when I was not invited to parties, sleepovers, or dates. Those early rejections created wounds that have followed me into my adult life. Of course, what wounds me today is couched a little differently. The circumstances and people vary. But the pain of those heart wounds—so real and raw—always led me to question my beauty and value.

I've spent years listening to women of all ages who often tell me the same kinds of stories I've experienced in my own life. I've been wounded by rejection, loneliness, grief, abuse, financial struggles, and fears for the future. The pain can feel too raw and too deep to overcome. Yet I've regained strength and hope with the Lord and true perspective.

Maybe you have felt the same way. Maybe you can identify with some of these struggles. Does the weight of daily life keep you in a stronghold of feeling unworthy and burdened with a list of to-do items that cannot be completed? Do you feel guilty about prioritizing yourself and your health? Do you struggle not to feel less than others when you compare your reflection with what you see on social media? Does it feel impossible to turn off the inner critic who constantly bombards you with negative messages about yourself and how you look or act? If so, you're not alone.

In preparing for this book, I asked two main questions to begin the conversations:

- *What obstacles do you face that prevent you from making lifestyle choices to improve your emotional or physical health?*

- *What bombards you daily to distract you from owning your true beauty? From experiencing health, hope, and vitality?*

As I settled in one evening to delve into the messages I had received from several women, I was reminded of how we are alike. We all want to be seen, heard, and truly known. We all want to feel beautiful inside and out, then stop worrying about it and move on with life, making a difference.

Many women described the obstacles they faced as a matter of logistics. They felt they lacked the time or were simply too busy and didn't have adequate support from those around them in pursuing their health goals. They were confused about mixed messages they would hear about what is healthy or unhealthy. Several women felt stressed. Many women didn't have adequate access to healthy foods or gym equipment, while others feared facing other people's judgments as they pursued their health goals.

But while logistics played a role, many women admitted that comparison was an even greater barrier to their health. The endless round of social media—with its unrealistic expectations, commercialism, photoshopped selfies, and surface image versus true identity—had eroded their confidence. As a result, they felt battered by the world's judgment rather than bolstered by God's love.

The answers I received to these questions are not that different from the messages I hear in my office from patients or when I speak at events. We tend to be our own worst critics.

Beautiful reader, I wish I could sit and discuss this face-to-face. I want all of us to begin each day by looking into the mirror and seeing our hearts and souls aligned with God. Then, we will be able to accept our present health status, surrendering what we cannot control but courageously owning our authentic beauty and reclaiming our health to steward our lives well.

The real beauty is that we are already seen, heard, and known. We are truly adored and unconditionally loved by our Creator. Let's take a deeper dive to consider some of the strongholds in our hearts and minds that hold us back from recognizing our authentic beauty and making lifestyle choices to care for ourselves with courage and grace.

Beauty in the Bible

Plans for one event had begun more than a year earlier, and now the day was fast approaching. Our team at WellSprings had decided to host a seminar for women of all ages to discuss the topic "Beauty for All Generations."

We wanted to encourage women to recognize beauty in every season and decade of life. The team had planned a day full of information on skincare, makeup, nutrition, and physical activity, along with door prizes, sales, music, and great food. Yet the most important part to us was the spiritual message we hoped to relay to the women, that we all are beautiful creations of the God Most High. In our inner circle, we called it the "Esther Event."

Woven throughout the entire day was the story of Esther. In the fifth century BC Persia, a young Jewish woman named Esther lived in the capital city of Susa. The Jews had been taken captive from Judah to Babylon by the Babylonians. The Persians defeated the Babylonians and took over the land and the people.

Cyrus, the ruler of Persia, had allowed some Jews to return to their homeland of Judah, but Esther stayed in Babylon. She was orphaned and raised in Persia by her cousin Mordecai, a strong Jewish man.

At this time, King Ahasuerus was in power in Susa. The king hosted a 180-day celebration ending with a 7-day banquet with the men while Queen Vashti, his wife, hosted the women. There was excessive consumption of food and drink throughout the event, and on the final day, the king asked his eunuchs to bring Queen Vashti into his banquet of men to show off her beauty. She refused! Advisors told the king he had to remove her as queen, or no man in the kingdom would be respected in his home. The king removed her from her royal position.

The king's advisors suggested doing a countrywide search for a new queen. They began to gather all the beautiful young virgins into the palace as a harem from which the king could choose a new queen. Esther was one of those women. Once the women were gathered, they began undergoing a twelve-month session of beauty treatments.

Esther's life and the extraordinary situation she encountered demonstrate how our circumstances don't define who we are or how we live our lives. Esther embraced and cared for her God-given, beautiful self despite hurdles and limitations. She displayed selfless courage. She gained the confidence and strength from God to face potential death by going in to see the king—uninvited—to ask him to save her people, the Jews.

When her cousin Mordecai reminded her of God's providence and provision for the Jews, he said, "And who knows whether you have not attained royalty for such a time as this?" (Esther 4:14).

Esther responded by asking the Jews to fast and pray along with her for three days. After that time, she would approach the king again. "And thus I will go in to the king, which is not according to the law; and if I perish, I perish," she bravely told Mordecai (Esther 4:16b). She demonstrated such trust and faithful courage.

I am reminded of Mother Teresa's quote, "I am not called to be successful; I am called to be faithful."[1] Let us lay aside the pressure to succeed according to worldly standards and instead seek to be faithful to our God-given purpose.

When I think of women of beauty in the Bible, Esther is the most obvious example. She embraced a ritual of twelve months of beauty treatments to enhance her God-given beauty before her introduction to the king. But many other women demonstrated beauty throughout scripture, as well:

- Abigail displayed resourcefulness, intelligence, and courage to protect her people and approach David to pursue peace despite the hard-hearted nature of her husband, Nabal.

- Mary, the sister of Martha and Lazarus, chose to pursue the most important thing.

- Mary, the mother of Jesus, endured challenges yet pondered and treasured all she witnessed.

Those are more obvious examples, but God directs our hearts and minds to find beauty in unexpected places:

- In Miriam, who served the Lord despite expressing fear, doubt, and even jealousy of her brother Moses.

- In Martha, who was distracted by the busyness of hospitality, yet was faithful to the Lord throughout his life and ministry.

- In Rahab, a harlot who chose God and protected His spies from the enemy, placing her own family in harm's way.

- And in the woman at the well, who listened and changed her life after spending a few moments with Jesus.

Past mistakes do not define any of us. What others say about us does not matter when matched by what God says about us. He knows our name. He affirms us.

"But you are a chosen race, a royal priesthood, a holy nation, a people for God's own possession, that you may proclaim the excellencies of Him who has called you out of darkness into His marvelous light" (1 Pet. 2:9).

God loves us beyond what we can fully understand.

"See how great a love the Father has bestowed upon us, that we should be called children of God; and such we are. For this reason the world does not know us, because it did not know Him" (1 John 3:1).

And no matter where we are in our journey of health, hope, and vitality, Jesus wants us. He desires to change us.

"For while we were still helpless, at the right time Christ died for the ungodly. . . . But God demonstrates His own love toward us, in that while we were yet sinners, Christ died for us" (Rom. 5:6, 8).

I believe true, authentic beauty rests in the deep recesses of our hearts, where God fosters what He has created. God will nurture that beauty and allow it to blossom outwardly.

Perfectly Created

As I prepare for work each morning, I look in the mirror multiple times as I go through my routine of showering, skincare, makeup, hair, and clothes. Those superficial, quick surface looks are important external daily checks that help me feel more confident. However, none of those glances focus on seeing who I truly am. They are important, but they do not define me.

My real look in the mirror—the intentional act of knowing and seeing myself beyond the superficial—occurs when I sit at my kitchen counter with hot tea, breakfast, and God's Word open for reading and reflection.

Some days, I am successful in making this happen, while other days, I am so rushed that I do not have that same time with the Lord. However, on those days, I strive to commune with Him as I go about my day. That is the beauty of God's truths. They settle into our hearts and minds and follow alongside us, whatever we do. Pausing and reflecting on God's truths and His love for us throughout our days will help us to remember that we are beautiful and free to live out of an authentically beautiful place.

We can easily get caught up in the world around us, navigating the day's demands and facing fear, struggle, comparison, and what-ifs. These are real needs that fall on us. But if we start our day by looking into the mirror of a heart filled with Him and choose to see our beauty, we will naturally radiate Him. Even as we walk through crazy, hectic days that sometimes knock us down and wound us, we can face each circumstance with a steady sense of joy and purpose. Our ability to possess that certainty begins with loving Him and loving ourselves.

Once we can look in our mirror and love the person we see because we see our Creator reflected in our image, we can move forward to love and encourage those around us.

For instance, few people like their nose, but it is the first place that air—breath, the spirit of life—enters our body. Our nose warms and humidifies the air. If you have ever visited Colorado and experienced its low humidity when it is cold, the nose has difficulty overcoming the rapid adjustment. The cold air can feel like ice picks in your lungs, and the dryness can even lead to nosebleeds. Our nose also allows us to smell and taste, with 80 percent of taste derived from our sense of smell. We can wear glasses and sunglasses thanks to our nose and ears. Trust me, your precious nose works hard to improve your life, so show it some love and appreciation.

Similarly, few people like their feet, but we should thank them for being strong and getting us places despite our abuse and neglect.

Try looking into your mirror and telling yourself these truths:

- *I love my smile because it may brighten someone else's day.*
- *I love my hands for allowing me to pick things up, hug people, and cook dinner.*
- *I love my legs, not for how they look but because they allow me to stand, walk, and release endorphins (the feel-good hormone).*

We are amazing, beautiful, strong, courageous women created by our awesome, sovereign God! Yet we usually look in the mirror and focus on our flaws. When we embrace the life-giving, soul-sustaining love of Jesus, we can walk away from our mirror in the morning and love others fully without comparison. We are made in the image of God, and when we find our worth in Him, all other comparisons begin to fade away.

A shift in our mindset is fundamental to owning our authentic beauty. The hurt, wounding, comparisons, and striving to measure up to the world's standard of beauty that is so entrenched in our culture hold us back from experiencing the free, abundant life God offers. Yet freedom from the bondage of cultural expectations really begins with a shift in our perspective. It begins with a change of focus. It begins with God and His Word and our decision to believe that our worth is clearly and completely defined by His unconditional love for us, not by ever-changing cultural standards. He created us. Choosing to shift our mindset results in a transformation in our hearts and minds. Yet this is only possible through our daily choices and decision to surrender, trusting that God's power will meet our desires and needs.

Despite our pain and wounding, we can choose how to respond. If we raise our eyes and look to God, He will guide us to acceptance, accountability, authenticity, and abundance. When we become grateful for all of our story—even the most difficult and painful parts—we will begin to experience His freedom. We know in the deepest recesses of our hearts that He redeems all of it for our freedom and His purpose and will. As we own the beautiful creation that we are, we can choose to claim our health. We have permission and are commissioned to take care of ourselves.

S N A P

Seek Him

Seek out His truths regarding your reflection in the mirror, then write your favorite scripture verses on cards to place beside your mirror to bring clarity to your beautiful reflection. You can either use some of the ones from this chapter or find your own verses that speak to you specifically.

Meditate on These Words

✞ For if you keep silent at this time, liberation and rescue will arise for the Jews from another place, and you and your father's house will perish. And who knows whether you have not attained royalty for such a time as this? Then Esther told them to reply to Mordecai, "Go, gather all of the Jews who are found in Susa, and fast for me; do not eat or drink for three days, night or day. I and my attendants also will fast in the same way. And then I will go in to the king, which is not in accordance with the law; and if I perish, I perish. (Esther 4:14–16)

✞ But we all, with unveiled face, beholding as in a mirror at the glory of the Lord, are being transformed into the same image from glory to glory, just as from the Lord, the Spirit. (2 Cor. 3:18)

☩ The Lord your God is in your midst, A victorious warrior. He will exult over you with joy, He will be quiet in His love, He will rejoice over you with shouts of joy. (Zeph. 3:17)

☩ For if anyone is a hearer of the word and not a doer, he is like a man who looks at his natural face in a mirror; for once he has looked at himself and gone away, he has immediately forgotten what kind of person he was. But one who has looked intently at the perfect law, the law of liberty, and abides by it, not having become a forgetful hearer but an effectual doer, this man will be blessed in what he does. (James 1:23–25)

☩ For now we see in a mirror dimly, but then face to face; now I know in part, but then I will know fully, just as I also have been fully known. But now faith, hope and love remain, these three; but the greatest of these is love. (1 Cor. 13:12–13)

☩ As in water a face reflects the face, so the heart of a person reflects the person. (Prov. 27:19 NASB)

Nourish Self

Nourish yourself with words of affirmation throughout your day. Find short little sayings or mantras that speak to your heart when the day's tumult tries to rob you of claiming your authentic beauty. You can write these on index cards attached to a ring clip, type them in your phone, use them as your screen saver, or post them around your home on small pieces of paper to happen upon during your daily routines.

- I was born worthy.
- I am loved by a sovereign God.
- My day will go according to how the corners of my mouth turn. (As you share your smile.)
- I am whole and complete.
- I have done this before, and I can do this again.
- I believe in myself and His power at work within me.
- I give myself unconditional love.
- I choose joy.

Armor of God

Trust that the armor you put on this morning when looking in the mirror can deflect any messages that come your way and negate your innate beauty, health, confidence, strength, or dignity. Some days feel more difficult than others. On those days, I get my armor on in a more demonstrative way. I look in my mirror and pretend to cinch down my breastplate of righteousness and belt of truth with an audible *Ca-ching!*

Prayer

Dear Lord,

As I reflect on Your unconditional love for me, help me to look in my mirror and see You reflected in me. Teach me to see what You see in me as Your daughter; help me to feel Your presence and provision. May I always seek to name what I am humbly grateful for in the person I see reflected at me. Thank You for the wisdom that I have gained from life. May I always embrace what the day has in store, trusting You to be with me, for me, behind me, and ahead of me. Allow the authentic beauty that I see to transform my heart and mind. Help me to move throughout the day filled up with You so that I can overflow with Your love, kindness, grace, and mercy to every person You place in my path. Help me claim my beauty and health and choose my well-being as I extend grace to myself.

In Your name,

Amen.

CHAPTER 2

Passion and Purpose

*W*E HAD JUST COMPLETED OUR MORNING PRAYER TIME at my dermatology office and were about to begin work for the day when one of the ladies answering the phones asked if she could add someone to an already overbooked schedule. She explained that the woman was very emotional when she called from the parking lot and wanted to be seen as a new patient.

She did not have an appointment but had been watching a mole changing on her skin for quite some time. Her father had passed away from melanoma, and feeling fearful about her mole, she felt paralyzed to schedule an appointment.

However, today was different. She had discovered the day before that she would be a grandmother in seven months and suddenly had a new reason to care for herself. I agreed to have her worked into the morning's schedule and went on to see the first two scheduled patients.

As I prepared to walk into the new patient's room a little later, I paused momentarily and thought about what motivates us to care for ourselves. Why do we need prompting for something to live for? Especially with skin cancer, early detection is critical to the outcome. What can I do to encourage patients not to delay a skin evaluation? What can I say to empower people to own their health and choose to prioritize it?

Those questions drive my passion for speaking to patients individually and at seminars about caring for themselves. I can offer a patient a prescription, surgery, or supplement to guide their treatment plan for a skin disease. However, my greatest impact is often in educating and encouraging them to understand how their lifestyle choices will impact their overall health and well-being, as well as the skin issue that prompted their visit.

This particular patient did have a cancerous mole on her skin. However, once I surgically removed the melanoma, the pathology report revealed that it was superficial and had a 99 percent cure rate with our wide local removal. She now gets regular skin examinations as part of preventative care of herself.

God is the source of our passion and purpose. Using the greatest commandment as our foundational answer to the questions of life, we are reminded to love. In three gospel accounts, Jesus reiterated to His followers and the Pharisees that we are to love God and our neighbors the same way we love ourselves. Yet our ability to love God and others will be determined by our choices to steward our spiritual, physical, and emotional health. Day by day, we can remove the obstacles that encumber us from recognizing our value and fulfilling our purpose. We can take baby steps to claim our health. We can choose to believe in our God-given beauty and live with confidence.

Stewardship of the bodies God has given us is not wrong. For followers of Christ, self-care is always others-centered and done ultimately for the benefit of those around us. It is just as necessary as putting on our own oxygen mask before assisting others in an airplane emergency.

This chapter sets the stage by focusing on our motivation to care for and steward our health.

Perfectly Created

Arriving at medical school on my third day of freshman year, I was filled with awe, fear, and anticipation. This was the day! A sacred day: The day we would be given access to a human cadaver we would work on for the entire semester. By utilizing the cadaver, we would become familiar with every single detail of anatomy underlying our deep intention to understand the body that we would spend our entire careers striving to help and heal.

My excitement rose as we were divided into teams of four and allowed to enter a room full of metal containers where we would be introduced to our work.

Until I was a medical student ready to start Gross Anatomy, I did not appreciate how perfectly created our bodies are to live in this world. We did not happen by chance. This semester-long course is one of the classes in medical school that one never forgets. The thrill that runs through every freshman medical student's veins when they are allowed to dissect a human body is a privilege beyond words. Visualizing how every muscle, tendon, bone, nerve, blood vessel, and organ works together is captivating and fascinating. Witnessing the intricacy of the human body also triggers a desire to take care of this amazing creation. In turn, this can also produce a desire to understand why God created us, what He intends for us to do in the world, and how we can fulfill His purpose.

God spoke us into existence, forming Adam from dust and Eve from Adam's rib. In an instant, this intricate, cell-based machine with an intelligent mind, spirit, and soul walked the earth and desired relationships and purpose. God could have designed our bodies any way that He chose. However, He designed us to require daily nourishment of food and water to fuel our cells. He gave us a mind with free will to decide how we would live and care for ourselves. You do not have to go to medical school to gain an appreciation and ownership of your body and health or to recognize how your choices impact your body. We can all choose to do this because we are children of God.

He has made each of us for a purpose, and we can live that out with our eyes on Him, not on the world. We truly are "fearfully and wonderfully made" (Ps. 139:14 NASB 1995). When we know and feel that truth to our core, we will not only radiate our authentic beauty but also never be a stumbling block for others to exude their beauty.

Yet our first step toward recognizing the gift of our bodies and reclaiming our health must be finding our *why*. It is vital for us to have a *why* to make any change in our lives.

My Why

I want people to understand and appreciate their purpose, own their choices, and enjoy health and vitality.

My why is formed partly due to personal reasons. First, as a mother to a generation who—for the first time in our country—has a lower life expectancy than their parents. Second, as a mentor to young people who live in a world with an all-time high incidence of teen anxiety, depression, addiction, and suicide. Third, as a daughter who cared for aging parents, which was a challenging journey. Some things impact our health that we cannot do anything about; however, we make many choices that directly affect our well-being. Our choices today will impact how we live the last five to ten years—those final years when our days can be filled with passion and purpose or appointments and pain. The quality of that life is decided now.

The final years of my parents' lives demonstrated that truth. My father, an esteemed general surgeon, spent the last several years of his life needing help with basic self-care. His health had deteriorated to the point that he could not do much at all. I spent time cleaning him up, shaving him, changing his clothes—all things that he had done for years for himself. Even as we spent his final years together, I prayed that my dad felt his "little girl" loving him well. He passed away in November 2019.

My mom (my most supportive cheerleader, most loyal confidante, my rock, and constant believer in me) worked as a math teacher, helped put my dad through medical school, collaborated with her parents to enlarge their grocery store into a hugely successful business, and eventually became the mayor of our city for eight years. Yet despite all those successes, her final years were marked by progressive dementia. Sometimes, she knew me and would interact with me, but her response was typically somewhat indifferent. Other times, she did not remember what I did or said from one minute to the next and sometimes even had fear, paranoia, and disdain in her eyes toward me. The change in our relationship was devastating. It was one of the most challenging times of my entire life. I prayed to God continually because when the pain became too difficult to bear, I begged Him to help me rise above my heartache of losing her—my real mom—and to let her *feel* loved by me. I prayed that she would continue to feel loved, appreciated, and admired.

This intimate close-up view—watching strong, intelligent, giving people live out the last few years of their life with pain, dementia, and limited opportunities—solidified in me a commitment to make choices now that will give me the best opportunity to live with robust health, hope, and vitality.

My why goes beyond my personal life, however. As a physician who has practiced medicine for thirty years, most days are filled with treating disease rather than bolstering health. Although I can provide an educated treatment plan, that is a small piece of healing. I see some patients who may know what needs to be done, while others require additional education about proper choices regarding food, exercise, stress, sleep, and supplementation. Yet, no matter how much knowledge or willpower they possess, living out healthy decisions can be challenging. Straight discipline or free will alone often only works for some people. Yet despite these obstacles, my desire to prevent disease remains. I remain committed to helping others live a life where health is owned, purpose is empowered, faith is solid, and hope is realized.

How can we determine our why? When it comes to our health, we must begin by asking ourselves:

- *What were our bodies made for?*
- *Why must they be nourished?*
- *How should they be sustained?*

Once we've answered those questions, we must consider the implications. Identifying our why is the first step, but understanding our resistance to change is also essential. What is our motivation to do anything in this life? Science demonstrates that we are more likely to stay committed to change when we know the reason behind the choice and the desired outcome is more clearly understood and visualized.

Human nature inherently drives us to seek comfort and gratification. Whether it is food, fun, or the perfect temperature in our homes and workplaces, we want to be comfortable. Yet what we want is only sometimes what is best for us in the long run.

You and I are facing an epidemic of instant gratification. It robs us of our potential and long-term goals. For instance, our brain may tell us that we want a dessert right now, yet we know that excessive amounts of sugar lead to increased inflammation and poor health—something none of us want. Succumbing to a choice simply because it's what we want in the moment will have long-term consequences.

It can sound defeating to hear that, as humans, we are naturally wired for immediate gratification. However, we can all be intentional about our choices. We can choose what is best for us. This intention, however, requires us to be self-aware of our tendencies and personal challenges. For instance, the life we have lived to the present puts a stamp in our hearts and minds that can leave us believing lies about ourselves and what we "need" to feel worthy, seen, known, valued, or loved.

How God Sees Us

If we take the time to start or begin again believing that we are worthy, special, and loved because of our Creator, then we are more likely to live with confidence and cultivate a desire to take care of ourselves so that we can love and serve others. This aligns with the truth of Proverbs 4:23 (NIV), "Above all else, guard your heart, for it is the wellspring of life." We must choose from our heart—the wellspring—not the world.

Think of your body as a strong and secure temple impacted by our external environment as well as the things that come into the innermost parts.

In 1 Corinthians 3:16–17 (NASB 1995), Paul says, "Do you not know that you are a temple of God and that the Spirit of God dwells in you? If any man destroys the temple of God, God will destroy him, for the temple of God is holy, and that is what you are." The Greek word for destroy here is *phtheiro* (see Strong's #5351), meaning to shrivel or wither, to pine or waste. Something shrivels or withers due to lack of use. Although this can be compared to our bodies and how we care for them, I believe Paul's main focus was in reference to the Lord's work. His point is that we must not think and live worldly lives, shrinking from telling others about our foundation in Jesus Christ. We are all created with inexplicable value, commanding honor and dignity.

Later in that same letter, Paul says, "Or do you not know that your body is a temple of the Holy Spirit who is in you, whom you have from God, and that you are not your own? For you have been bought with a price: therefore glorify God in your body" (1 Cor. 6:19–20). Paul reminds readers to glorify God in our bodies with everything we do, say, or think.

Considering these two points, we must recognize that our physical health means nothing if we lack spiritual health. However, we can only live out what He has created us to accomplish with our physical health intact. That, ladies, is what we *must* own! Be deliberate about your habits. Just like physical workouts, our spiritual habits help us grow. They go hand in hand. Let's not "default" in either area of our health.

Many women tell me that they want to lose weight. I encourage them to explore that desire. If this is your desire, ask yourself:

- *Why do I want to lose weight?*
- *What is my ultimate goal?*

The answers to these questions can be vast, varied, and fluid. For instance, we can desire to lose weight because we believe it will make us more attractive or "better." Or perhaps our motivation to change is rooted in shame imposed by self or others regarding our appearance. It can be due to a recent diagnosis that accelerates a smoldering desire to optimize our health. Or it can be deeply rooted in our desire to be more effective in our daily calling.

Our motivation—our why—must start in our hearts. This conviction becomes more personal and ultimately leads to freedom from the heavy weight of rules.

The renewal of our minds—the transformation—then follows. It is *how* we make a change in our lives. The *how* of a goal like this is secondary and must come after the *why* and *what* are established.

I do not intend to oversimplify the reason to choose yourself and your health, nor am I implying that recognizing your authentic beauty is as simple as stating it aloud. However, it starts there, and it ends there. I encourage you to say the following verse as often as needed to keep the junk messages that try to sabotage and complicate this truth from taking hold:

"For it was you who created my inward parts; you knit me together in my mother's womb. I praise you, for I am fearfully and wonderfully made" (Ps. 139:13–14 NRSV).

Please do not just read over these words because they are familiar. Take a moment to join me in that Gross Anatomy class. Let's sit together in awe, wonder, and amazement. Pause to reflect on the fact that our lungs expand and collapse, inhaling and exhaling air without us consciously telling them to do that. Consider how our gut and intestines use enzymes to take the food we have eaten and convert it to fuel to run our brain, muscles, and individual cells to do the work they were created to do. We are a true wonder, each one of us! All of us collectively!

It does not matter what season of life you are presently in or what your health looks like. Choose you. Choose that place between guilt and regret, and value yourself. Love yourself so that you can love others.

In the following chapters, we will educate and encourage ourselves toward excellence in wellness and beauty for the glory of God, thereby equipping and empowering us to impact others. We will learn about lifestyle choices that allow us to be our best selves. And we will begin by recognizing and owning our authentic beauty. From that place of self-acceptance, we can define our why and commit to choosing life.

Moving Forward

The rest of the book will walk you through practical ways to claim your health through nutrition, exercise, social media, relationships, words, skincare, and finding joy. Yet, along the way, I want you to find encouragement to understand that this is not a list of rules to follow. This is a journey of freedom, self-forgiveness, and fun.

We will learn to set goals. We will accept that we can follow those goals while extending grace to ourselves. We can be steadfast in following through with these alone, but finding accountability partners who are loyal and trustworthy can help make the journey so much more colorful.

Let's not wait to find the "perfect" checklist, app, or diet—simply choose what works for you and will support you from a health and well-being standpoint, then move on.

The stress of regret or rethinking a "bad decision" in food, lack of exercise, etc., is as much of a problem for your health due to the stress hormone cortisol release as the "poor choice," so make your choices and live with freedom.

I have read many books that inspired, encouraged, and informed me. I hope this book will help you realize you own many of your health choices, if not most. I want you to feel me alongside you, seeing your authentically beautiful self, living out the one precious life God has given you, just as I hope to be doing the same.

It does not matter where you are in your health journey; simply make the next best choice to choose *you*. Each step will allow you to move toward health, hope, and vitality. So, start. You can do that. You can believe in yourself. We are never the victim but always the victor in Jesus.

I encourage you to begin by exploring the habits, tendencies, and default choices that may need to be modified or even totally changed in your life. Then, begin to journal and write down some goals you want to pursue and steps to reach them. This exercise can be repeated for all areas of your health and well-being. Just as there is a physical component to our health, there is a spiritual or inner component as well.

Authentic beauty starts from within. It is then nurtured throughout experiences, decades, and seasons of life. Finally, it is lived out as a gift to others, all while God is glorified. When we focus on steps to take and choices to care for ourselves in the midst of a busy life, we expand from victim to victor, from self alone to self *and* others, from within to without. This is the freedom that abundant living provides.

We can all begin to balance making healthy choices by surrendering to the transformation that God will do in our lives.

S N A P

Seek Him

Many scriptures focus on following God and His will for our lives. Although there is much debate about how we can truly know God's will, I believe the more time we spend seeking to know God, the more likely we are to be led by the Holy Spirit and live by the Word.

Meditate on These Words

✞ For my thoughts are not your thoughts, nor are your ways my ways, declares the Lord. For as the heavens are higher than the earth, so are my ways higher than your ways and my thoughts than your thoughts. (Isa. 55:8–9 ESV)

✞ The heart of man plans his ways, but the Lord establishes his steps. (Prov. 16:9)

✞ Delight yourself in the Lord, and he will give you the desires of your heart. (Ps. 37:4)

✞ You will seek me and find me, when you seek me with all your heart. (Jer. 29:13)

✝ Be very careful, then, how you live—not as unwise but as wise, making the most of every opportunity, because the days are evil. Therefore do not be foolish, but understand what the Lord's will is. (Eph. 5:15–17 NIV)

✝ Trust in the Lord with all your heart and lean not on your own understanding; in all your ways submit to him, and he will make your paths straight. (Prov. 3:5–6)

✝ The thief comes only to steal and kill and destroy; I have come that they may have life, and have it to the full. (John 10:10)

✝ Let no debt remain outstanding, except the continuing debt to love one another, for whoever loves others has fulfilled the law. (Rom. 13:8)

Nourish Self

Find some time to sit and write down what you value in life. Explore what innately brings you joy when setting long and short-term goals.

What do you enjoy doing in your free time?

Who is a priority to you?

Write down what brings you joy and hope: The relationships, accomplishments, possessions, and activities that mean the most.

Make a chart with each of these above categories and ponder the why for it and the desired outcome purposed by that desire. Write whatever comes into your mind about steps you can take today, next month, and next year to spend your time in this life guided by your heart's true desires. Color-code the chart to make it more fun and focused. Find a fun, useful calendar or planner to keep you accountable.

Revisit this chart monthly.

Armor of God

Time is such a precious commodity. We cannot add to it. However, we can use it for those things that are most valuable to us. So let's be intentional about choosing how and where to spend our time.

As the saying goes, "If you fail to plan, you are planning to fail." Today, write down intentions and boundaries you can set to help you prioritize the most important things. Include meaningful and helpful boundaries in your plan that are realistic or work for you so that what you deem as most important or most connected to your passion is given time and space to flourish. That will permit your purpose to be first and foremost in your mind, heart, and calendar.

1. Book a monthly meeting with yourself. Set aside a small amount of time every month to review your calendar and commitments and begin to edit. Just as in the Netflix show *Get Organized with The Home Edit*, we accumulate items and activities on our calendar that are no longer a priority and, therefore, have not earned a place in our lives right now. Fix yourself a cup of hot tea, open your calendar, and ask God to guide your edits as you prioritize your time and schedule.

None of us can do it all. As Anne Lamott says, "'No' is a complete sentence."[1] Some really good things end up on the "editing floor," as the movie editors say. Permit yourself to cut some things out so you can show up more focused in life with your true passions and purpose. This will look different in different seasons of life, which is okay.

2. Hold your calendar with open hands and heart to accept God's direction and guidance. There will always be times when we must set aside our plans and pivot our attention due to things that arise in life. It is often best to have built-in flexibility in your calendar, and I encourage everyone not to overbook or completely book their days. Warren Buffet once said that he keeps his calendar open for whatever may come up within a day.[2]

3. Put it into practice. Once you've determined your priorities and commitments, get a calendar—either paper or digital—and begin to fill in blocks of time:

   - Time with the Lord
   - Time to plan and schedule my week
   - Time for fun, work, and family
   - Time monthly to re-evaluate where my time is spent and what needs to be adjusted

   Finally, set a reminder on your phone to prompt you to have a date with your calendar, start with prayer, and trust God to guide you.

Prayer

DEAR HEAVENLY FATHER,

*Y*OU CREATED ME AS I AM, WITH MY SPECIFIC AND UNIQUE characteristics, and You love me! I desire to honor You with this beautiful, precious life. As I walk through the days and weeks ahead, give me the focus and discipline to set boundaries and intentions for my time, decisions, goals, and choices. I do not seek a check-off list of dos and don'ts but a heart committed to You and You alone. Please help me strive to know and hear You above all of the distractions of this world. Help me grasp in the deepest recesses of my heart the way You see all of me—the flaws, regrets, mistakes, failures, hurts, and longings—and use them all for Your glory and honor.

Guide my life so that it truly is a life that matters!

In Jesus's name,

Amen.

CHAPTER 3

Best-Kept Food Secrets

*S*EVERAL YEARS AGO, I WAS IN AN EXAM ROOM WITH A four-year-old patient discussing treatment options for his atopic dermatitis (a skin disease with scaly red patches of skin that itch and are uncomfortable) with his mother. I asked her what type of diet he consumed. She quickly corrected me, letting me know he was not on a diet. *Hmm?*

Well, actually, diet is simply a reflection of the foods we eat. This word has been taken hostage by a culture obsessed with diet in the context of losing weight. So we must reclaim the understanding that we typically choose what, when, and how we eat, which defines our diet. I am not a fan of camping out in a media-driven category of diets. The goal should be to eat real food, mostly vegetables—beans, legumes, grains, and fruits.

The number on a scale does not define *anything* about our beauty or worth. Neither does size, clothing, hair length, or hair color. However, choosing what to fuel our bodies with is critical. This one temple—this one body—is all we have to fulfill our God-given calling. So, we must honor this temple by being faithful stewards of our health choices.

It's a myth that healthy eating is too difficult or too expensive. It is all about choosing and embracing the foods that our bodies were made for so that we live lighter, less encumbered, more vibrant lives.

Unpacking Our Feelings on Food

Like our understanding of diet, food is another four-letter word that controls us if we let it. For many years, I struggled with a flawed understanding of health and how my food choices impacted it.

My personal health story changed dramatically in 2000 when I faced two health crises. Within three months, I was diagnosed with pancreatitis requiring sphincterotomy (a disease where the digestive enzymes of the pancreas that are released to help digest food were backing up and destroying my pancreas due to a scarred duct from gallstones) and ulcerative colitis (a disease with inflammation, ulceration of the colon).

As a result, I had to learn which foods wouldn't cause pain and would instead help me to remain the active mother I wanted to be. I already ate a fairly healthy diet but had never fully learned about the SAD (Standard American Diet) or how some companies in the food industry put profit over people and produced an inferior quality of food or used inaccurate messaging in advertising and packaging.

Back in the 1940s, people often ate what they grew in their gardens, supplementing with products from the grocery store that they couldn't grow themselves. But due to convenience, shelf life, and productivity, the Standard American Diet eventually moved from being supplemented by products to relying on them as the primary food source. Unfortunately, processed foods are not simply food. They also include chemicals, preservatives, and ingredients our bodies do not recognize. They are not absorbed well and lead to inflammation. They also potentially contain bacteria, fungi, hormones, and antibiotics, which affect our microbiome.

Our organs require nutrients from our food to function. Digestion is the process that occurs in our gastrointestinal system to take the foods that we eat, utilizing enzymes and microorganisms that inhabit the lining of our gut (microbiome) and allowing these nutrients to be absorbed through the lining of our GI system into our blood vessels to be carried throughout our body and then utilized for optimum function of our organs. Our food quality dictates the microbiome's health, the ratio of usable nutrients, and our overall health.

The foods we eat are one of the most significant influences on the amount of inflammation in the body. Eating foods that promote inflammation (refined carbohydrates like white bread, fried foods, soda and other sugary beverages, red meat, processed meat, and dairy) causes free radicals to form, which damages the cells in our body. Inflammation wreaks havoc on our body in almost every way and must be minimized to optimize our health. Eating "anti-inflammatory" foods—such as colorful vegetables and fruits—can protect us from these harmful effects.

My own health difficulties sparked a journey of studying nutrition and foods and discovering the nuances of food choices. Even though I am a doctor, medical school historically does not teach nutrition and its impact on our health, and many physicians have not been trained to understand its complexity. If nutrition is complex for someone who works to understand the human body every day, it's no wonder it might be confusing for the average consumer. So trust yourself as you seek out reliable and accurate information. Begin to explore and make some changes for yourself. If you want to become more aware of how foods impact your body, keeping a diary for several months of the foods you eat and how you feel after eating them can be helpful. (See the SNAP portion of this chapter for how to get started.)

Yet regardless of how much we know (or don't) about proper nutrition, we all need to eat—and our food choices will impact our long-term health. Not everyone will receive the diagnosis I did, but many other diseases have been linked to insufficient fruits, vegetables, beans, legumes, and grains. As a doctor, I'm concerned that arthritis, stroke, fatigue, foggy brain, cancer, heart disease, kidney stones, ADD/ADHD, Alzheimer's, dementia, anxiety, skin disease, and dental disease are not only lurking but are also now linked to food. We have come to accept many of these as normal aging, but that is not the case.

The truth is that our understanding of foods and what they do in our bodies is continually evolving. We are learning more about the enzymatic and cellular levels of digestion every decade.

Over the years, I've encountered several patients whose experiences demonstrated the link between nutrition and overall health. One woman came to me as a new patient after battling psoriasis vulgaris for years. Psoriasis vulgaris is a skin disease composed of thick, itchy plaques on the skin. Although inherited, it has variable penetrance, which means it will manifest differently for different people. Some people may carry the gene and never have any skin rash, while others have plaques in the most common areas of the scalp, elbow, knees, and lower back. However, it can even become widespread over the entire body. This patient had recalcitrant plaques on her shins, arms, and scalp that were uncomfortable and made her very self-conscious. Though she had been on systemic treatments of pills and injections as well as topical prescription creams, they had improved the skin but not cleared it.

This condition is very important to treat, not only because of the cosmetic and comfort concerns but also because several comorbidities align with active psoriasis. In other words, people with continued systemic inflammation that keeps psoriasis active also have an increased risk of arthritis, depression, inflammatory bowel disease, and cardiovascular disease. All of these are related to unchecked chronic systemic inflammation.

Knowing all of that, I explained the role of inflammation to my patient. I told her that she could improve her psoriasis and lower her risk of these other diseases later in life by making lifestyle choices and changes. She listened attentively and left empowered to do her part. She avoided dairy, artificial sweeteners, and soda, and she also decreased her sugar consumption. She began to read labels and recognize that even when a product is labeled "sugar-free" or "zero sugar," it can include four to six chemical sugars that are even more damaging than regular sugar.

Six weeks later, she returned to the office. By then, her psoriasis had cleared. Within six months, she was off all her topical and systemic medications.

This is a beautiful story of someone willing to listen, learn, and make some changes in her choices, and her health improved. However, many patients struggle to adapt their diet to support their health. As discussed in chapter 2, defining our why—our desire to make healthy food choices—can help us change our mindset about food. We begin to understand and consider food as fuel to enjoy a healthy, energetic life. When our mindset shifts, the food choices we make follow almost effortlessly. Food, meals, and fellowship around the table are vital to life and health. Yet, in this fast-paced world, we often eat on the go, mindlessly consuming calories but not getting nourished. So pausing and deliberately considering how and why our body requires food can alter our choices. For instance, if we think we need coffee, carbohydrates, or sugar to energize us when we are tired, then that is what we will reach for when we are sluggish. If we think our energy level or focus is low because we are dehydrated or undernourished, we will reach for water and real food such as a salad, quinoa, beans, apple, nut butter, avocado, carrots, or hummus. Changing the purpose of food in our minds—so that we eat to live with energy rather than to satisfy hunger from lack of proper nutrition—will translate into overall improved health.

Food isn't simply fuel, however. Fellowship around the table—breaking bread and consuming meals together—is one of the greatest gifts of eating. Whenever it is possible to sit down at a table and eat with friends, loved ones, or new acquaintances, then laughter, learning, and love will follow. In fact, the National Center on Addiction and Substance Abuse at Columbia University found that children who ate meals together as a family five to seven times a week were more likely to perform well in school and were significantly less likely to smoke, drink alcohol, or use illicit drugs.[1] There is such a gift in time together that goes beyond the actual nourishment of our bodies. We experience a greater sense of purpose and value when our souls are fed as well. It reminds me of when my three children were growing up. Whenever we sat down to dinner, we asked each other what the "bummer" of the day was and the "highlight." One powerful result was our ability to see and understand each other more authentically.

Although I enjoy working with adults, I absolutely love teenagers! In fact, the youngest of my three children told me during his senior year of high school that one of the ways he felt loved by me was whenever someone said to me how difficult teenagers were or how they dreaded the teen years with their kids, I responded by saying that I loved and cherished every stage. Each age is delightful and challenging, but that is the beauty of staying present and connected to our kids as we guide them through those changing times in their minds, bodies, and spirits.

So, when a teenager comes to see me about acne, I love to lean in and get to know them. One Tuesday morning, as I paused before entering Exam Room 1, my medical assistant filled me in on a new patient. She was fifteen and struggled with acne on her face, back, and shoulders. She had not used any prescription medications but had tried multiple over-the-counter acne treatments that had not helped much. When I opened the door, I was met with beautiful yet questioning eyes. This young lady sat nervously, fidgeting on the exam table. Her mother sat attentively in the chair to the side.

I wanted to let her know that I saw her, desired to know her, and would do my part to help her skin heal and become healthier. So, after some pleasantries, I listened as she shared what bothered her the most about breaking out and all the things she had tried. I then asked her to share what she knew about acne and prescription acne treatments from social media because there is a lot of information out there. Unfortunately, much of it is inaccurate, but it helps me know where we are starting our education. I reassured her that I was older than Google, so she could trust me!

Next, I moved on to our plan of action. I reviewed the three critical steps to establishing skin health (cleansing and toning twice daily and using a scrub twice a week) before adding any prescription medications and the "why" behind them. We then discussed the prescriptions I recommended for her particular acne. She listened attentively as I described the process occurring on the skin on a cellular level, including our expectations and approach to keratin cells. Her keratin cells needed to be exfoliated for us to improve her acne, but for three weeks, that exfoliation may be perceived as dryness. However, I urged her only to use the moisturizer I recommended because many of them sit on the skin and lock keratin cells back onto the pores, negating what we can achieve with our treatment plan.

Then, I addressed food and its impact on acne. She looked devastated when I told her about foods that worsen acne because they promote inflammation, including dairy, soda, artificial sweeteners, sugar, and chicken. She looked at me squarely and said, "That is all I eat. I eat mac and cheese and a soda or diet soda at least one meal a day. I love pizza, cheeseburgers, and ice cream. I will just die if I have to give them up!"

I smiled softly, reassured her that she would not die, and reminded her that these changes were her choice. When she returned for her first follow-up, she told me she had followed the skin treatment plan without making any food changes. Although her skin was better, it was not clear. She was frustrated and wanted her skin to be clear before school started in the fall a few months later. I offered her some documentaries to watch and websites to glean even more information about foods and inflammation.

At her subsequent follow-up, she was clear from acne, had radiant skin, and said her body had never felt better than it had since making those food changes.

Recently, I had a similar conversation with another family. I discussed the importance of eating whole foods, and they said I was destroying the joy of eating. What a disheartening way to look at nourishment! We need to pause and rebrand how we consider food.

I gently reminded them that I was not taking the joy out of food. God put vibrant colors and flavors in foods and spices; a quick look at a farmer's market or produce section reveals our wide variety of options. Look at the bountiful colors! A fun way to explore flavors is to choose a fruit or vegetable that is new to you or that you have not tasted in a while. Buy it, and then cook, eat, and enjoy it. Let the whole process be life-giving, not life-depleting.

Our bodies are fueled by our food choices, and we can experience a change in our health trajectory by changing the narrative in our minds about foods. I encourage you to be willing to spend some time learning about this with an open mind and a willing spirit. Doing so is beneficial in many ways, including an increase in confidence. Knowledge is power, and understanding how our food choices impact our short- and long-term health is the first step in giving us the confidence to keep moving toward health.

What the Bible Says about Food

Before we unpack the science of food and our current understanding of the best way to support our health through our food choices, we must consider God as the original source of wisdom.

After all, God—our Creator—could have created our mortal bodies however He desired. Yet, He made us depend on food to refuel our cells to function, repair, be healthy, and survive. Why is that? What purpose does food have in our lives? Why are we forced to pause in our day and partake of food?

God created us to be intelligent beings, and we can choose for ourselves what to consume. But how do we know what or how God intends for us to eat? Interestingly, scripture has some things to say about our choices.

In Genesis 1, the very first chapter of the Bible—God's inspired Word—we read the account of God's creation of the heavens, the earth, and everything in them. At the very end of that chapter, in verses 29–31, God says,

> Behold, I have given you every plant yielding seed that is on the surface of all the earth, and every tree which has fruit yielding seed; it shall be food for you; and to every beast of the earth and to every bird of the sky and to every thing that moves on the earth which has life, I have given every green plant for food, and it was so. And God saw all that He had made and behold, it was very good. And there was evening and there was morning, the sixth day. (NASB 1995)

God desired and designed us to consume plants and seeds from the very beginning. He made many different varieties for us to eat. Our bodies were created to be fueled with lots of fruits and vegetables, seeds, and grains.

Then again, in Daniel, we read the story of Daniel and his friends, Hananiah, Mishael, and Azariah. In his interactions with the commander of the officials, Daniel requested that he and his friends be allowed to eat a certain way for ten days:

> But Daniel made up his mind that he would not defile himself with the king's choice food or with the wine

which he drank; so he sought permission from the commander of the officials that he might not defile himself. Now God granted Daniel favor and compassion in the sight of the commander of the officials, and the commander of the officials said to Daniel, "I am afraid of my lord the king, who has appointed your food and your drink; for why should he see your faces looking more haggard than the youths who are your own age? Then you would make me forfeit my head to the king." But Daniel said to the overseer whom the commander of the officials had appointed over Daniel, Hananiah, Mishael and Azariah, "Please test your servants for ten days and let us be given some vegetables to eat and water to drink. Then let our appearance be observed in your presence, and the appearance of the youths who are eating the king's choice food; and deal with your servants according to what you see." So he listened to them in this matter and tested them for ten days. And at the end days their appearance seemed better and they were healthier than all the youths who had been eating the king's choice food. So the overseer continued to withhold their choice food and the wine they were to drink, and kept them eating vegetables. (Dan. 1:8–16)

Though they chose to eat differently than the king and his officials, they were healthier and had an improved appearance. What some may have seen as a sacrifice or self-denial was a blessing and gift to their health and countenance. Like Daniel, we can make choices that may feel difficult at the moment but will foster long-term health. When we pause and change the narrative on how we choose our foods, we can make intentional decisions to support our health and promote vitality.

Though these passages were written long ago, they continue to have implications for us today. So much information about our health comes from the internet and other sources that distract us from trusting the age-old reality that our bodies need real food—they always have and always will.

I like how author Sheri Rose Shepherd discusses the connection between the spiritual and the physical:

> My Beloved Daughter, Your body is My dwelling place: the place My Holy Spirit resides. My greatest desire is for you to experience good health in your spirit and in your body. Spiritual war will not be won if you go to battle exhausted and weak, My beloved. Take time, My love, to rest and rebuild my temple, your body. I have prepared a table for you to feast from My Whole Foods. If you commit your diet to Me as My prophet Daniel did, I will reward you with favor, strength, and wisdom, just as I did for Daniel during his reign. Now is your time to do what is needed to run your race and finish strong![2]

We can choose to be intentional about our food and develop the resilience to abandon mindless eating altogether. I find it interesting that God made us dependent on food and water as a life source. We must continue to return to food for nourishment. But it is also interesting that food was the downfall, the vehicle used to bring sin into this world. When Adam and Eve were in the Garden of Eden, they were free to eat all the plants and trees in the garden, except for the Tree of Knowledge of

Good and Evil. The enemy enticed Eve and manipulated her ego, leading her to eat from the forbidden tree. That act of eating the forbidden fruit is what brought sin into the world. Similarly, our food choices can protect our health and prevent disease *or* promote and enhance disease.

A woman in her early fifties who is a counselor and therapist wrote this to me when reflecting on her declining health situation. She said,

> Several years ago, I read a book called *God Loves Ugly* by Christa Black. The author wrote a statement that has always stuck with me. "Your body is a house, and that house provides a means of carrying around the most precious cargo in the universe: you."[3] Well, my house has been really messy for about a year now, and it's time I cleaned it up.
>
> First Corinthians 6:13–15, 19–20 is quite implicit about this. I cannot begin to tell you how these words seep into my soul and cause me unrest. I have given God my soul but kept my physical body to myself, mistreating it, criticizing it, and neglecting it. But God thinks I am beautiful. So beautiful, in fact, that He died for me! (2 Cor. 5:17). I proclaim in the name of Jesus Christ that I am ready to make a change. I will no longer use food as a substitute for the Holy Spirit. I will use food for fuel, thankful to God for sustaining me each day. I will learn to love myself so I can fully love others and receive the love others give me. I am ready. If you are ready to change your life, start by surrendering to God and embracing the new life that has come.

This woman discovered that making changes and surrendering to God brought freedom from the many mixed messages she'd received from others and herself. Her story can become your story. Her freedom came by making better choices and extending grace for the occasional not-so-good choice. But, for all of us, our first step toward freedom begins when we decide to pay attention and steward our choices rather than default to what we know. God desires this kind of stewardship in our lives, and He is glorified in us when we follow through.

As she mentioned, Corinthians discusses how our body is a temple for the Lord:

> Food is for the stomach, and the stomach is for food; but God will do away with both of them. Yet the body is not for immorality, but for the Lord; and the Lord is for the body. Now God has not only raised the Lord but will also raise us up through His power. Do you not know that your bodies are members of Christ? Shall I then take away the members of Christ and make them members of a prostitute? May it never be! . . . Or do you not know that your body is a temple of the Holy Spirit who is in you, whom you have from God, and that you are not your own? For you have been bought with a price: therefore glorify God in your body. (1 Cor. 6:13–15, 19–20)

Most of us have seen a temple. In the Old Testament, a temple was a place where God dwelled. It was a structure that housed His presence, and the priests were tasked with maintaining the temple. In the New Testament, after the death, burial, and resurrection of Jesus, all of God's people became His dwelling place. As Peter wrote in 1 Peter 2:5, "You also, as living stones, are being built up as a spiritual house for a holy priesthood, to offer up spiritual sacrifices acceptable to God through Jesus Christ." In a way, we are now tasked with caring for ourselves, the inner parts of our outer being, where we are His dwelling place. We are to work and conserve ourselves for His service.

Our diet—the foods that we eat—are choices. We usually choose what we eat and drink and must recognize our responsibility. This journey is not about being perfect. It is not about eating to look a certain way, wearing a particular size, or seeing a number on the scale. Instead, it's about choosing health for long-term vitality. It is choosing to honor and glorify God as we show Him our gratitude for our health and our God-created masterpieces—our body, soul, spirit, and mind.

The Science of Nutrition

My husband, a head and neck surgeon, and I have both experienced how challenging it can be to convince people they can hold off on undergoing surgery or taking a prescription to improve their disease by changing their lifestyle. They often opt for surgery or pills, even though these options carry potential risks and side effects. I understand how daunting life changes can feel and how taking a pill can seem simpler (and honestly is at the moment), which is why I'm passionate about helping people see that nutrition need not be difficult. I have walked this road. I truly understand the daily and sometimes hourly "restrictions" that weigh on us as we try to make changes. But trust me, it is worth it!

I recently noted someone's T-shirt and had to stop and ask for a photo. Though it was meant to be humorous, I was struck by its message about the impact of multiple medications on our overall health as we chase the side effects of other medicines by adding more. The shirt read:

> I take metformin for diabetes caused by the hydrochlorothiazide I take for high blood pressure, which I got from the Ambien I take for insomnia caused by the Xanax I take for the anxiety that I got from the Wellbutrin I take for chronic fatigue, which I got from the Lipitor I take because I have high cholesterol because a healthy diet and exercise are just too much trouble.

Medications serve a purpose and can be beneficial; however, I challenge all of us to reconsider their role in our long-term health plan. Instead of relying on them to fix everything that ails us, what if we considered them short-term protections for our health as we work to make healthier long-term lifestyle choices? Over time, as we make thoughtful decisions regarding food, exercise, stress management, and sleep, we may find that our bodies require less medication than they once did.

Our goal should be to increase our health span, not merely our lifespan, and we can use food to promote vitality and longevity as another kind of "medicine." As Hippocrates said in 440 BC, "Let food be thy medicine and let thy medicine be food."[4]

One of the reasons I love chatting with patients about lifestyle changes is because I've seen firsthand how much they can help. For instance, atopic dermatitis is a skin disease that starts early in children and is often associated with allergies and asthma. Signs of this condition can arise as itchy, scaly patches, particularly in the folds of the skin—such as the inside of elbows, behind the knees, in the axilla, and around the neck—but can occur on the whole body. Often, topical medications can control the rash and symptoms, but sometimes, we must consider more aggressive but effective treatments, including regular shots of immune-modulating medications.

As a physician, I am grateful for the medical advancements that bring healing and relief to my patients. I am continually reading the literature and appreciate the research and development in my area of professional training because it helps me care for all of my patients more effectively. Yet science has also shown that this disease process is driven by inflammation; therefore, any lifestyle changes—notably in food choices—that a patient can make will help the disease tremendously. Since many of these patients are children, I start by discussing the importance of avoiding inflammatory foods as well as first-, second-, or third-hand smoke with the parents. I am saddened by how frequently parents will balk at food changes they see as "depriving" their child and instead default to giving them a shot when those food changes would often render the shot unnecessary.

All of us are impacted by the foods we eat. One of the most empowering advancements in medical research is in the area of genetics, specifically nutrigenetics. We used to believe our genes were just our cross to bear or our blessing to enjoy. We have good genes, bad genes, cancer genes, obesity and diabetes genes, etc. However, we have discovered that the foods we eat can turn those genes on or off. Even better, across the board, all disease states are improved by the same selection of foods. Eating real food—like a variety of fruits and vegetables along with beans, legumes, and grains—improves our overall health, helps to prevent chronic disease, and turns off the harmful genes most of us have inherited. There is not one diet that is good for heart disease, one for the kidneys, one for fighting cancer, another for the skin, another for the lungs, liver, teeth, etc. All systems in our body improve and function at their best with a daily intake of nine to thirteen servings of various fruits and vegetables.[5]

The problem is that less than 12 percent of children and less than 10 percent of adults in the US consume this amount.[6]

So what are we going to do about this discrepancy? Thankfully, we can do our part to improve those statistics by increasing our own fruit and vegetable intake. This helps us, but it is also an example for all eyes watching us. Here are a few simple tips to keep in mind:

- Aim to include nine to thirteen servings of a variety of fruits and vegetables every day to optimize health and prevent disease.

- We used to believe that plaque in arteries was permanent. Now, we know we can decrease plaque by increasing fruits and vegetables, similar to how we descale our coffee machines.

- If dealing with stress, exercise, or chronic disease, increase that to seventeen to nineteen servings daily. However, it is very challenging to get that on our own. One strategy is incorporating a plant powder supplementation, which can bridge the gap with thirty servings of fruits and vegetables daily. Backed by more than forty medical journal articles, this strategy is my "insurance" to ensure I receive the necessary servings of fruits and vegetables to optimize health and prevent disease. I have chosen to partner with the one company, Juice Plus, that does this and has proven research plus pays a third party for NSF certification (testing each batch to confirm that what is on the label is actually in the product and nothing else). Juice Plus is a food supplement. It is real food, dehydrated, and put in capsules or gummies.

- Plant-based eating is also becoming more common, making it easier to include more fruits and vegetables in daily food choices.

- Get most of your protein from beans, legumes, and grains.

As the science and understanding of nutrition and its impact on health evolve, so does the food industry. The food industry collectively focuses on profitability and production, which can negatively impact the quality of the food. The food industry will use commercials and ads to entice us with appealing visuals. Food labels are helpful but can be misleading. For example, potassium bromate is often added to flour that is used in bread, rolls, cookies, and other baked goods "to make the dough rise higher and give it a white glow," even though the International Agency for Research on Cancer considers it a possible human carcinogen and its use has been banned in Europe.[7] The bottom line is to be a wise consumer by educating yourself and remembering that this field will change and adapt.

Advancements in agriculture, distribution, shelf-life for processed foods, convenience foods, eating out, and genetically modified foods for higher production and longer viability will not change the fact that our bodies function best by consuming cleanly grown and harvested food. But despite the conflicting messages we hear, we can choose what we listen to and believe. The newest or latest in food, skin care, or exercise is not always better. Take the time to find trustworthy and reliable sources for your health information.

Food can seem complicated, and it often is, because there are so many levels of depth to how food reacts in our bodies, including understanding micronutrients (enzymes, vitamins, and minerals) and macronutrients (proteins, carbohydrates, and fats). But we can make it easy for all by simplifying what we know.

For instance, it's a myth that healthy eating and drinking are more expensive. Drinking water from our faucets is free, which is much cheaper than purchasing flavored packets mostly made of chemicals to put in our water, sugary sodas, or other drinks. Removing processed and unhealthy snack foods from our grocery carts and instead spending most of our food budget on fruits, vegetables, grains, and beans will save money. When we shop the periphery of the grocery store—buying unprocessed, real foods—we will decrease our food budget over time. Doing so will also support our health, setting us up to save on future healthcare costs.

After all, food is our building block and the source from which our cells, brain, muscles, organs, bones, hair, skin, and nails gain energy, vitality, and the ability to function and repair. Choosing food that supports our bodies is one way to help foster long-term health.

As consumers, we can do the work to know what we are eating. It's our prerogative to decide if quality is more important than quantity and assumed cost. For example, even though a McDonald's burger and french fries may be cheaper than buying a salad, the temporary "savings" may be deferred to later in life, costing us more when our health eventually suffers due to poor nutrition. It's important to recognize how the cost of poor health can also manifest itself as lost income, lost experiences, diminished quality of life, and lost opportunities to serve God and others—when we are sick or don't feel well, it's hard to do more than the bare minimum.

Yet there *is* hope. It is never too late to change our health trajectory.

I have multiple patients every day tell me there is no way they can give up processed foods they love, like mac and cheese, ice cream, soda, diet drinks, artificial sweeteners in their coffee, coffee creamer, sugary foods, and other foods and beverages that promote inflammation and lead to disease. I understand that it's hard to feel like we're giving something up, but the truth is that we're gaining something much more important—our health. Prioritizing short-term satisfaction over long-term health gives food too much power. We must eat to live, not the reverse.

Here are some simple tips to help you down the path toward healthy eating:

- Eat from the periphery of the grocery store, focusing on fresh fruits and vegetables.

- Google how to cook new things. (Not fried items, however.)

- Natural foods straight from the earth are the healthiest. Daniel provides a wonderful biblical example of this type of eating.

- You are more likely to remember what you research yourself. However, use reputable sources like nutritionfacts.org.

- Visit a farmers' market. If you have children, let them choose a vegetable or fruit to take home. (Bonus points if they help cook or prepare it in the kitchen!)

- Consider joining a CSA (community-supported agriculture). Purchasing a half or whole share will provide fresh, local fruits and vegetables during the growing season.

The food we eat begins with what we purchase, whether at the store or a restaurant. When you buy packaged foods, read the labels. Google questions like: *What is a healthy ingredient on a food label? How much sodium and sugar should I consume?*

As your meal plan for the week ahead, consider these additional tips:

- Minimize animal protein and let that be fish or quality red meat.

- Increase plant protein with sources such as beans, grains, quinoa, nuts, and seeds.

- Avoid toxins, processed foods, packaged foods, and salt.

- Limit sugar intake, which can spike insulin levels, increase inflammation, and is often accompanied by brain fog. (Some restaurants have even started putting 30 percent sugar in their saltshakers.)

- Avoid artificial sweeteners. (Many are known carcinogens.)

- For some people, avoid gluten and wheat.

- Avoid or minimize dairy, which includes milk, yogurt, cheese, and ice cream. Dairy is an inflammatory food.

Despite longheld beliefs, we do not need dairy as a source of calcium. We consume enough calcium in our vegetable intake to maintain proper bone health, especially if we avoid soda, which depletes calcium from our bones.

- Stop drinking sodas, sugary drinks, all drinks with artificial sweeteners, or beverages with the words "diet," "zero," etc. Save your health and your money by drinking water. As my urology colleagues say, our urine should be clear, not yellow. Several factors determine our need for hydration, including salt intake and sweating, so in deciding how much water to drink, I advise patients to consume enough water so that their urine is almost always clear.

- Avoid chicken due to widespread contaminants, hormones, and antibiotics.

As you consider each day's meals, here's a quick visual of what your plate should look like:

- Half of the plate should be fruits and vegetables.

- One-fourth should be carbohydrates such as rice, quinoa, sweet potato, and blue potatoes.

- One-fourth should be protein, such as beans or a small portion of meat (3 ounces). Protein requirements have been misleading for quite a while. Most of us only need about 40–50 grams of protein a day (0.8 grams of protein/kg/day). Too much protein can lead to bone and calcium balance disorders, impair renal or liver function, increase cancer risk, and precipitate the progression of coronary artery disease.

- Monitor your portion sizes. Think before you eat: *I do not need to clean my plate.* Eat until you are 80 percent full, and then stop. The stretch receptors on your stomach take a few minutes to notify you that you have had enough, so stop early. (Using smaller plates may help reinforce smaller portions.)

- Quantity over quality is not real value. So do not fall into the enticement of "supersizing" a meal.

Although these tips may feel daunting initially, they'll become second nature over time. As noted above, begin by visualizing your plate and embracing the narrative of prioritizing your health.

Truly, every day I am in the office, I see patients who could feel better and improve their skin by simply changing the foods they consume. Most of the time, we do not connect our foods to how we feel. Yet we can be wise, discerning, and thoughtful in our food choices and have *fun* learning to try new things. Doing so has changed my life!

S N A P

Seek Him

Inhale, Exhale, Pause . . .

This chapter is full of information about food. I ask that you keep an open mind and seek God's guidance in striving to eat with the ultimate goal of caring for your God-given temple.

Meditate on These Words

✝ You also, as living stones, are being built up as a spiritual house for a holy priesthood, to offer up spiritual sacrifices acceptable to God through Jesus Christ. (1 Pet. 2:5)

✝ Give thanks to the Lord, for He is good, For His lovingkindness is everlasting. . . . Who gives food to all flesh, For His lovingkindness is everlasting. (Ps. 136:1, 25)

✝ If you consent and obey, you will eat the best of the land. (Isa. 1:19)

✠ Do not work for the food which perishes, but for the food which endures to eternal life, which the Son of Man will give to you, for on Him the Father, God, has set His seal. (John 6:27)

✠ But He answered and said, "It is written, 'MAN SHALL NOT LIVE ON BREAD ALONE, BUT ON EVERY WORD THAT PROCEEDS OUT OF THE MOUTH OF GOD.'" (Matt. 4:4)

✠ Better is a dish of vegetables where love is, Than a fattened ox served with hatred. (Prov. 15:17)

✠ It is not good to eat much honey, nor is it glory to search out one's own glory. (Prov. 25:27)

✠ Food is for the stomach and the stomach is for food, but God will do away with both of them. Yet the body is not for immorality, but for the Lord, and the Lord is for the body. (1 Cor. 6:13)

Nourish Self

Activity 1: Keep a nutrition journal.

Try keeping a nutrition journal for three months. Write down what you eat and when you eat it. Write down how you felt throughout the day at the end of each evening. Consider recording how your energy level changed (if you felt bloated or heavy or focused and energetic versus sluggish and tired).

Pay attention to how your body feels after eating certain foods.

For instance, we can eat a meal with quite a bit of dairy and afterward have stomach cramping, bloating, or generally feel unwell. We can eat a meal with more sodium and end up with a headache and cotton mouth. We can eat a meal of heavy animal protein or saturated fat from another source and feel sluggish and fatigued. We can consume high amounts of sugar in a drink or food and feel anxious for a short time, then too tired to do anything—leading to more sugar or caffeine.

On the other hand, we can drink water throughout the day so that our urine stays clear in color, and we have a more focused mind and energized body.

We can consume a rainbow of fruits and vegetables throughout our day and notice sustained energy.

After thirty days, what conclusions did you draw? What foods made you feel the best? Which ones made you feel the worst? Did you decide to make any changes based on what the journal revealed?

Now, continue for another sixty days, stopping to gain clarity at the end of the next thirty days. Everyone's body will respond differently to certain foods, so become aware of your body and what helps you feel your best.

Activity 2: Read and respond.

The Blue Zones contain the highest concentrations of functional centenarians in the world. These long-lived individuals have several characteristics in common: Most eat local, plant-based diets, with lots of beans utilized as the plant protein and animal protein only consumed about once a week. They exercise using daily movement. Many stay connected socially and honor their ancestors, and 97 percent are faith-based individuals. Most of these people eschew retirement, choosing to live with activity and purpose throughout their lives. These individuals are not trying to live longer; it is just their way of life.

How can we utilize the Blue Zones information to help us make better choices throughout our lives? Here are a few tips for every season of life:

- Teens/20s: We can get away with poor eating choices for a while. However, the combination of synthetic hormones in our standard American diet (which leads to earlier puberty), increased sugar (leading to increased anxiety), filler, and toxins will impact the body over time. The good news is that now is a great time to learn how to cook and get creative with food to establish healthy habits.

- 30–50s: A busy calendar filled with our families, careers, or communities tends to define our choices. Try meal planning and prepping beforehand to avoid eating foods simply because they are convenient. However, remember not to shame yourself or feel guilty when you do not have time to plan ahead. Move on, desiring to make the best choices when you can.

- 60s and older: Make sure to get enough protein. People tend to eat less, so pack in nutrient-dense foods. Don't quit moving. Cook and mentor others in their own healthy eating journeys.[8]

Considering the information above, what are two actionable steps you can take this week to support your health based on your age?

Are you interested in learning more? The Blue Zones website (www.bluezones.com) provides a wealth of information, including articles, recipes, and a weekly newsletter.

Additional Resources

Documentaries:

- *What the Health*
- *Forks Over Knives*
- *Super Size Me*

Books:

- *Your Body in Balance: The News Science of Food, Hormones, and Health* by Neal D. Barnard, MD
- *The Blue Zones Solution: Eating and Living Like the World's Healthiest People* by Dan Buettner
- *Codependent No More: How to Stop Controlling Others and Start Caring for Yourself* by Melody Beattie
- *Deadly Emotions: Understand the Mind-Body-Soul Connection That Can Heal or Destroy You* by Don Colbert, MD

Websites:

- www.nutritionfacts.org
- www.forksoverknives.com
- www.plantricianproject.org
- dremjones.juiceplus.com
- dremjones.towergarden.com

Armor of God

Our daily food requirement reflects our need to go to God daily for spiritual food—His Word—seeking His Spirit and guiding light for our life. Food also reminds us to pause and experience friends, families, and coworkers through socialization.

When we begin a lifestyle change, like rethinking our food choices, we must use intention and energy to help us focus and make good decisions. Therefore, as you begin this journey, say some of the scriptures written above every morning. Write them on cards that you keep with you. Bookmark them in your phone to remind you.

Take pictures of healthy, colorful food as a reminder of the beautiful options that God has provided for us and keep them in the photo reel of your phone or on a Pinterest board you look at often. Fall in love with the beauty of real food, not processed or packaged foods.

Those images will be armor for your mind and body as you choose healthy and life-giving foods.

Prayer

DEAR HEAVENLY FATHER,

YOUR WISDOM IN CREATING OUR BODIES IN SUCH AN intricate way—allowing us health, function, and vitality as Your masterpiece—is humbling. You alone could design the many facets of our anatomy and physiology.

Thank You for Your bountiful creation, providing such beautiful, tasty, nourishing foods. Guide me in choosing foods that will nourish me in a way that optimizes my health and prevents as much disease as possible. Give me the vision to make difficult choices in the moment of hunger so I can live a long, active life of service for You.

Put people in my path who will encourage and empower me to take care of this precious temple You have given me for my life. Then, allow me to mentor others on better stewarding our food choices.

When I am confused about what is best, please grant me wisdom to proceed with discernment.

In Jesus's name,

Amen.

CHAPTER 4

Strengthen Yourself for God's Calling

A FEW YEARS AGO, I ATTENDED THE ANNUAL CHAMBER of Commerce dinner in our hometown with about three thousand people in attendance. The guest speaker, Vallie Collins, was a passenger on US Airways Flight 1549, which landed on the Hudson River on January 15, 2009.

Though many passengers saw their life's memories flash before them, Vallie couldn't help but focus on all she would miss. The experience influenced her views on kindness, empathy, perspective, and time, but it also helped her realize how important it was to be physically fit.

Standing on the wing of the slowly sinking plane in freezing cold temperatures, preparing to climb on a raft for safety, she encountered a young mother holding an infant and toddler. The mother was in shock, frozen in place, and unable to move or help her children. Vallie had to get the two children, the mother, and herself into the raft. She then had to help them scale a rope-style ladder to the ferry waiting to rescue them.

That mother and her children depended on Vallie and her strength and agility to get them all up that ladder to safety. The moment helped her realize that we never know what will be required of us to help others survive, and being fit can make a difference, just like it may determine how effectively we can fulfill our God-given purpose.

The Lord calls us over and over to care for ourselves. As Proverbs 31:17 reminds us, "She girds herself with strength and makes her arms strong." The Lord desires us to stay physically strong as women of God. God gave us physical bodies to help meet physical needs. This chapter provides examples of incorporating movement and strength into our everyday lives.

Turning Obstacles to Exercise into Opportunities

There has never been a period in my life when I had more time than I had ways I desired to spend it! My life has been busy for as far back as I can remember. In the past, exercise has been one of the first habits to fall off of my to-do list. I struggle to ensure it stays a priority because life pulls me to things that feel more important and urgent. However, exercise is one of the few things that keeps me feeling my best. When I have experienced seasons where I did not exercise, my body started hurting, my mind and anxious thoughts escalated, peace took a backseat to worry and restlessness, and my interactions with others were negatively affected. From forcing myself to stop studying and go to an aerobics class in medical school to parking further away from the door at the grocery store and maneuvering young children into the building to get more steps in, I have had to figure out ways to move my body intentionally. We all must look at our obstacles as opportunities to find innovative ways to exercise and add movement to our day. As the Blue Zones Solution checklist reminds us, we must "de-convenience" our lives so that we are forced to move more, not less.[1]

There will be seasons when finding any time to carve out as intentional workout time is impossible. When our calendar is full of school or work, we have young children at home, are running a taxi service for school-aged children, or are caring for aging parents, then we can accept that this is a season of life. We can adjust our expectations accordingly to do our best, and that is okay. However, regardless of the season, we can remain empowered to care for ourselves. We are more likely to stay the course if we focus on health over convenience and acknowledge that exercise will differ depending on our season and age.

Acknowledging the difficulties of our current season is an important first step, but it's not the only obstacle we face. Several women have shared with me that they feel inundated by others needing them. Just when they think they will have time to get back on track with their fitness goals, questions, phone calls, text messages, and others' needs bombard them to the point where they feel unable to breathe.

One woman told me, "I think some of my struggle is a conflict of desires. I want to be a good Christian, wife, and mama— and I want to like how I look. Sometimes, I think those conflict with each other because of the amount of time each requires."

While this is definitely true, it does not have to be paralyzing. Let's think outside the box to find something that will work for us in each season of life. Consider listening to scripture on audio, a podcast, or uplifting Christian music while exercising, walking, or cleaning. Multitasking can be detrimental to our sense of focus. However, this combination of listening to something while doing a routine physical or cleaning task is synergistic and beneficial.

Another woman in her fifties told me, "I felt as though, even if I were to focus hard on my physical health, I could really never measure up to the culture's standards of beauty. There were seasons in my life when it didn't seem worth the effort or otherwise felt very vain."

Consider negating the culture by quoting scripture about how beautifully God has made you and tuning out those voices. Look into exercise and movement that makes you feel good and is enjoyable! Remember, the internet and your phone are yours. Put boundaries on the information and voices that have access to you so that the messages you hear are encouraging. Own your phone, and do not let it own you! Silence the noise.

Although it is vital that we check in with ourselves to ensure our exercise or physical health commitments are health-focused rather than ego-driven, prioritizing our health can lead to increased joy and energy, which can help us in other areas of life that matter to us.

Some women have shared that fear paralyzes them from proper physical health stewardship. They fear growing older, failing, not being smart enough, or giving up their life to care for others. Remember that fear is not from the Lord. As Philippians 4:13 reminds us, "I can do all things through Him who strengthens me." So let go of fear. Find people who can guide you to exercise wisely and own your health that way. Many times in my life, I have sought advice from a physical trainer, physical therapist, yoga instructor, or exercise enthusiast to help guide me and get me on track, finding weekly movement that fits that particular season of life. Remember, none of us are born knowing these things. I am a physician and understand our bodies' anatomy and physiology, but I am not an exercise expert. So I have personally found people to help me navigate how to lift weights to keep my muscles, posture, and core healthy and in proper alignment.

Other women know how to support their bodies and realize they need to get some physical exercise regularly; however, they struggle with self-control. It may even feel easier not to start.

I am fortunate that my day-to-day work requires me to stand and walk all day. I rarely sit down. When I attend a conference, sitting down all day for lectures feels brutal. But for people with desk jobs or sedentary daily routines, you may have to find creative ways to add more movement. Consider a standing desk to use while working. Get up hourly and walk around, take a few steps, do some standing push-ups on the countertop, or incorporate walking lunges into cooking dinner.

One sobering statistic in the US is that 80 percent of adults and adolescents are insufficiently active. Only 18 percent of adult women and 12 percent of high school girls meet aerobic and muscle strength guidelines. This lack of activity is expensive, not only for our long-term health but for the US healthcare system: $117 billion in annual healthcare costs and about 10 percent of premature mortality are associated with inadequate physical activity.[2]

A more accurate perspective on this is to force ourselves to acknowledge that choosing not to exercise or incorporate movement in our days now will have consequences later. This decision will often determine how the last ten to twenty years of our lives are spent. Not everything is within our control, but our choices can influence the amount of pain, freedom, abundance, vitality, passion, and purpose we experience. Physical activity fosters normal growth and development and can make people feel, function, and sleep better. It also reduces the risk of many chronic diseases.

What do we do when our spouse or significant other does not support our pursuit of better health? What do we do when we need more time or resources?

Although there is no right answer to these challenges, we can find alternative solutions. Perhaps that requires finding an accountability partner—a neighbor to walk around the neighborhood with us, a friend who attends the same gym, or a fellow mom who brainstorms with us for healthy eating and exercise habits while we watch our children play soccer together—to help us stay consistent.

It is also crucial to extend grace to ourselves. Too often, we set a rigid goal of exercise that is honestly not sustainable. Then, when we fall short and have a few days or weeks where we do not follow our plan, we get stuck and quit.

When that happens, we must return to our why. Why do we want to be healthy? How will exercising help us achieve greater energy and vitality? With those goals in mind, why not start caring for our bodies each day by moving and strengthening them?

Mental health and physical health are very closely linked. As the Physical Activity Guidelines for Americans notes, our mental health, cognitive function and reasoning, sleep, anxiety, and depression are all improved by physical activity.[3] Though prioritizing our health through exercise can be difficult to incorporate into our schedule, its positive effects will spill over into other areas of life.

Finding What Works for Us

One of the issues I often hear from women is that daily physical exercise feels impossible. However, physical movement throughout the day is—by definition—physical exercise. Let's redefine how we see tasks like weeding the yard or vacuuming the stairs. We can impact many muscles through regular activity throughout our day.

Watches and Fitbits can be helpful tools that remind us to get up and move. It truly can be as simple as that. Getting up and moving every hour for a few minutes can positively impact our health.

Years ago, I was appointed by the governor of our state to the Get Healthy Kentucky Initiative. The main focus for those two years was to research what could be done in our school systems to improve overall childhood health during the school day. One of the exercise kinesiologists who spoke with us emphasized research demonstrating how children learn better, focus intentionally, and retain more information when they move five minutes every hour.[4] As a result, we recommended that each teacher be provided with a "Fit Deck" card set for their room, and at the beginning of each class or hour, they turn one card over and have the entire class perform that movement or exercise for five minutes. We can all do this. It is such a simple concept, yet it is backed by research and science.

The good news is that we don't have to make changes without help. I remember the first time that I met with a trainer to learn how to lift weights. I chose to go to a very small women-only gym and meet with a trainer. I was very intimidated on my first day. I had only spoken with the female trainer on the phone beforehand. I planned to work out three days a week for thirty minutes on my lunch break between seeing patients.

That morning, I felt inadequate packing workout clothes to change into before I went to the gym. I grabbed a collection of mismatched athletic pants, a top, socks, and tennis shoes. A thought entered my mind: *If I had a new, maybe matching or coordinated outfit, I would look more the part when she met me. Maybe I would feel more confident, capable, and ready.* But the only clothes that would have fit that bill were slick, leftover '80s jogging suits that my kids would have been mortified to see me wear. So I took what I had and went to work.

All morning, between seeing patients, I felt increasingly nervous about the gym visit ahead. *Would I be able to do what she wanted me to do? Could she help me get stronger? Would I know less coming in than anyone else she had ever trained?*

Finally, it was time. I finished my morning patients, quickly changed clothes, filled my water bottle, and headed to the gym. She greeted me with the obligatory paperwork.

Then, she sat down across from me and thoroughly assessed my health, limitations, and past exercise history. She immediately made me feel comfortable. She was fit to the core. Beautiful in appearance. Quiet in her demeanor. Confident in her words and actions.

I struggled with the first exercise she asked me to do and started laughing at myself, telling her I was sure anyone else could do this particular exercise better than me. I felt weak and inadequate. She calmly said, "You are doing great. Trust yourself. I've got you." I thought she probably could not relate to my weakness because I was sure she had been fit her entire life. When I said those words aloud, she shared part of her story with me. She told me that was simply not the case at all. She had struggled with weight and fatigue, yet one moment of driving around the Walmart parking lot changed her life. She was trying to find a closer parking spot to decrease how far she would have to walk to get into the store and realized, "I am too young for this. Something must change." It did. *She* did. Now, she is helping others do the same, including me.

Some women can feel intimidated by physical exercise. This includes cardiovascular work, such as walking, running or cycling; weight training; stretching; or balance work, such as yoga.

Find what works for you in the season you are presently in, using the community resources that are available to you. Many community gyms have trainers who will get you started on a workout routine. Reach out to people you know to see if they will partner with you to keep you accountable. Find local yoga classes and sign up for a beginner class. Go to the park and find out what others are doing. Swing on the swing sets. Take up tennis, golf, pickleball, or any other sport that brings you joy and community. Be willing to ask for help! Remember, none of us are born knowing everything about exercise, so jump in wherever you are and start moving. Curiosity will benefit you alongside all of the sweet little eyes watching you. It's okay to look silly or unsure.

One of the ways that I elevate my heart rate is by playing Nertz in the office with my nurses in the middle of the day. We eat lunch, clear off the table, push our chairs out of the way, stand up, and let the energy begin. We all feel better after simply twenty minutes of standing, actively playing cards, and laughing together in our own competitive way. Or we take the stairs a few times or play a game of ping-pong. Just move!

If you need a little extra boost, remember that our physical training can positively relate to spiritual training. I love this encouragement from 1 Corinthians 9:24–27:

> Do you not know that those who run in a race all run,
> but only one receives the prize? Run in such a way
> that you may win. And everyone who competes in the
> games exercises self-control in all things. They then
> do it to receive a perishable wreath, but we an imper-
> ishable. Therefore I run in such a way, as not without
> aim; I box in such a way, as not beating the air; but

I buffet my body and make it my slave, lest possibly, after I have preached to others, I myself should be disqualified.

Remember that no matter what your exercise journey has looked like up until now, you can begin again every week by adding more intentional and functional movement into your life. You can start to strengthen and empower your muscles to work for you to live an abundant life of vitality.

SNAP

Seek Him

Wherever you are on your journey of physical movement and exercise, give yourself grace and acceptance so that you can step out of your comfort zone to try something new. Make sure you continually stay in the Word of God, increasing your awareness of your motivation behind any new exercise. Doing so will help you steward your health and stay strong and full of vitality rather than focusing on looking a certain way.

MEDITATE ON THESE WORDS

✝ She sets about her work vigorously; her arms are strong for her tasks. (Prov. 31:17 NIV)

✝ Therefore, I urge you, brothers and sisters, in view of God's mercy, to offer your bodies as a living sacrifice, holy and pleasing to God—this is your true and proper worship. (Rom. 12:1)

✝ Therefore I do not run like someone running aimlessly; I do not fight like a boxer beating the air. No, I strike a blow to my body and make it my slave so that after I have preached to others, I myself will not be disqualified for the prize. (1 Cor. 9:26–27)

✟ So whether you eat or drink or whatever you do, do it all for the glory of God. (1 Cor. 10:31)

✟ But those who hope in the LORD will renew their strength. They will soar on wings like eagles; they will run and not grow weary, they will walk and not be faint. (Isa. 40:31)

✟ For physical training is of some value, but godliness has value for all things, holding promise for both the present life and the life to come. (1 Tim. 4:8)

Nourish Self

Activity 1: Take our survey: How much exercise is "enough"? Circle the stage of life you're in and write out a weekly exercise plan.

Exercise at every age:

- 3–5 years old: Physically active throughout the day to enhance growth and development.

- 6–17 years old: Daily 60 minutes or more of moderate to vigorous physical activity.

- Adults: At least 150–300 minutes/week of moderate intensity or 75–150 minutes/week of vigorous, intense aerobic physical activity or an equivalent combination of the two. Include muscle strengthening two or more days/week.

- Older Adults: Multicomponent physical activity that includes balance training, aerobic, and muscle-strengthening activities.

- Pregnant/post-partum: At least 150 minutes of moderate-intensity aerobic activity/week.

- Adults with chronic conditions or disabilities: Follow key guidelines when able.

What does moderate or vigorous intensity mean? Try the "talk test":

- Moderate: Can talk but not sing.

- Vigorous: Can only say a few words without pausing for a breath.

Defining different types of exercise:

- Aerobic: Endurance or cardio. Large muscles move in a rhythmic manner for a sustained period. Increases heart rate; breathing is more labored. Examples: Walking, brisk walking, running, cycling, and swimming.

- Muscle-strengthening: Resistance and weight training. This is important because our muscles hold and support our joints and posture. This type of exercise causes the body's muscles to work or hold against an applied force or weight. Examples: Use elastic bands or body weight to work on all major muscle groups, including legs, hips, back, abdomen, chest, shoulder, and arms.

- Bone-strengthening: Weight-bearing or weight-loading. This produces a force on the bones of the body that promotes bone growth and strength.

- Balance activities: Improves the ability to resist forces within or outside the body that cause falls while a person is stationary or moving. It also improves by strengthening back, abdomen, and leg muscles.

- Stretching: Dancing, yoga, tai chi, gardening.

For example, here's my own routine. Despite some of my own health challenges (scoliosis, ulcerative colitis, stress, neck compression from a car wreck, pancreatitis) and honestly, because of it, I choose to discipline myself in the following areas:

- Weight training with a trainer twice a week
- Yoga (two to three times a week)
- Cycling (two to three) times a week
- Foam rolling/stretching daily

Activity 2: Move your body.

Even small amounts of exercise and movement make a difference and positively impact our physical and mental health. Look for ways to add new movement to your life throughout your day.

- Take the stairs instead of the elevator whenever you can.
- Keep walking shoes with you in case the opportunity arises to squeeze in a walk.
- Park father away from the doors when running errands.
- When the weather gets colder, keep jackets, hats, and gloves available so you can still get outside and move.
- Try new outdoor games such as cornhole or four square.
- Have impromptu evening dance parties or stretch or do yoga while watching a TV program you enjoy.

Armor of God

Now write down the intentions and boundaries you can set to help you prioritize the most important things. The different components of our spiritual armor can reflect our commitment to physical movement.

Find the truth (Eph. 6:14) about exercise by seeking knowledgeable and trained professionals to help you get started and progress safely and effectively.

Protect your heart as you contemplate the "right" reasons for exercise (Eph. 6:14). Your aim should be to care for all aspects of your muscles, strength, flexibility, core, posture, and balance to remain functional throughout your life.

Ephesians 6:15 reminds us to be firm-footed and grounded in the gospel, which is foundationally a place of peace. This description is metaphorical but can also be literal: Our exercise journey does not need to feel like drudgery but can instead be enjoyable, full of peaceful curiosity, joy, and fun. Let's extend grace to ourselves when we let seasons pass by without staying diligent, even as we recognize that that sense of commitment will render sustained peace.

Hold on to your shield (Eph. 6:16) to bring perspective on your "why" and keep Satan from hijacking this stewardship, leading to an unhealthy focus on body image.

Keep salvation always in your mind as you focus on stewarding this life well, yet know our bodies will be whole in our true home, Heaven.

Above all, measure all that you do with the Word of God.

Prayer

DEAR HEAVENLY FATHER,

I PRAISE YOU FOR MY BEAUTIFULLY AND WONDERFULLY made body and the intricate design of muscles, organs, ligaments, joints, nerves, and blood vessels, all made by You.

Grant me the wisdom to show gratitude daily for my health. Help me appreciate how my arms and legs allow me to walk, hug, move, and serve others. Give me the understanding as to how my eyesight, hearing, sense of touch, and smell are all from You.

Help me to make the time to care for my body in a way that provides strength and lack of pain. Put people in my path who can guide, teach, and encourage me as I strive to stay accountable to myself and You.

Help me to see that there are pockets of time spent doing mindless things that do not improve my walk with You and that I can reclaim that time with daily steps to exercise and strengthen my body.

In Jesus's name,

Amen.

CHAPTER 5

Social Media Is Not Social Connection

*S*everal years ago, I decided to do some educational television commercials about skin health. One day, I went to the local television station with several outfits and four scripts to tape all four commercials. I was nervous but pleased with the results once they let me do a few practice takes to get used to the teleprompter. The commercials' messaging was effective.

But about two weeks after the commercials started running on air, one of my management team members told me she wanted me to hear a message someone had left on her voicemail. We walked into her office after I finished my day of seeing patients, and she played the message aloud for both of us to hear. The message shocked me; I still remember the tone, words, and humiliation I felt as I listened to the voicemail. The caller said she was so disgusted by the sweater I wore for one of the commercials that she could not even hear what I had to say. She said that if I had no better fashion sense than to wear an outdated argyle sweater, I surely was not up to date with dermatology treatments. She criticized my entire staff for allowing me to wear such a hideous fashion ensemble on air.

I wish I could tell you that her words did not get past my ears before I dismissed them. I wish I could say that at my age and in my position, I could laugh her comments off as nonsense. But I was honestly crushed. I went home that evening and removed that sweater from my closet to give to a local charity. I did not make another commercial for a few years. She won for a while. She won until I decided that I could choose what voices I listened to and allowed into my mind.

Why do we let other voices, many times from people we do not even know, impact how we feel about ourselves? Why do we let others control how we show up? What happens inside our heads and hearts when we are criticized or bullied when we put our true selves out there through social media, speaking, or writing?

The truth is that you and I can put ourselves out in public with healthy boundaries—whether that's through TV, radio, social media, blog posts, or other writing—and gauge our feedback through the lens of what the Lord says about us. We can lean into our loyal confidantes, ask for their opinions, and let the rest fall on deaf ears.

Relationships are vital to our lives, well-being, and work for the Lord. We all crave the social connection that comes from spending time together, leaning in, and being curious. Unfortunately, many have categorized social media or other online relationships as social connections, but those avenues cannot replace real relationships.

Statistics illustrate how teenage depression, addiction, and suicide are at an all-time high. According to the CDC, in 2021, 42 percent of students felt persistently sad or hopeless, and nearly one-third (29 percent) experienced poor mental health. In that same year, 22 percent of students seriously considered attempting suicide, and one in ten attempted suicide.[1] While these statistics are sobering, even for adults, bullying, fear, and anger are pervasive in our country and culture. And the continual bombardment of messages we receive that everyone else has a "perfect selfie life" is a critical catalyst for this disease. All too often, the connection we seek online falls short of our expectations, leading us to feel even more lonely and isolated.

This loneliness can have a powerful impact on our health and happiness. One study published in the journal *PLOS Medicine* noted that "loneliness has such far-reaching consequences that the health impact is comparable to smoking up to fifteen cigarettes a day."[2] While many of us have grown well-versed in the dangers of smoking, we're less inclined to take loneliness as the serious risk it is. However, loneliness is not only associated with an increased risk of heart disease, depression, and cognitive decline, but social isolation in seniors carries additional risks, including chronic health conditions, dementia, and early mortality.[3]

How can we engage with others online or in the public sphere without losing the in-person connections that help us fend off loneliness? Let's work together to learn how to embrace the beauty of social media while tossing aside the comparison/guilt cycle. We can learn to avoid absorbing negativity while committing to authenticity. Let's set boundaries on these distractions and gain more confidence, time, and perspective.

Social Media and Our Mental Health

Though the statistics are sobering, the personal stories I hear from women about social media and its sometimes detrimental effect on them amplify those concerns. For instance, when I asked a woman in her late twenties what bombarded her daily to distract her from owning her beauty, she quickly identified the source without reservation:

Social media and screen time. [Seeing others'] highlight reel and letting myself lose vision of what truly matters in life. I have to take regular breaks from social media because I am guilty of letting myself feel "less than" after seeing my stories and my feed. Social media influences so much of what I think I should look like or what I think I should be doing to be successful in life. Beauty, fashion, things, trends, trips, date nights, hanging out with friends, workouts, what I ate today, educational degrees, opinions, etc. Goodness, how overwhelming to keep up! Social media can also become a place that makes me feel like everything I do or say is wrong because I might be offending someone else.

It can be easy for us to fall into the comparison trap, and women of all ages are recognizing the impact of social media on themselves and those around them. As a woman in her late fifties told me,

Women are constantly comparing and basing their self-worth on other women. Everyone has to be a size 0, or they are overweight. Television, magazines, and social media now decide what's perfect; if you aren't, you aren't valuable. I work in a high school filled with young ladies with no self-worth. I was that girl; I can relate. Jesus is the only hope.

Comparison is a continual theme when I speak to women of all ages. Everyone is tired of the comparison game. They feel shackled by the relentless pursuit of something other than who they are or what they have.

Let's stop trying to measure up. Let's drop the pretense, posing, performing, and perfectionism that enslaves us. True "soul"-cial wellness begins with asking God to show us areas in our relationship with Him that need improvement, understanding ourselves better, and becoming filled up and overflowing with grace toward others. Instead of trying to inform others of their faults or ignoring our troubles, let's make our own decisions prayerfully and allow other women to do the same.

It's crucial to ensure that God's voice—and His love for us, His beautiful creation—isn't drowned out by social media voices that try to tell us otherwise.

After all, as Galatians 5:1 reminds us, "It is for freedom that Christ has set us free. Stand firm, then, and do not let yourselves be burdened again by a yoke of slavery." We can choose freedom; part of that is determining who or what we listen to. When we mindlessly scroll social media, we can become immersed in the world's constant heartache and violence displayed on our feeds. Immersing ourselves in this kind of negativity robs us of peace and contentment and paralyzes us from living out the purpose right in front of us. We can only do so much. We cannot impact or alleviate every sorrow and loss the world faces, and setting boundaries or filtering out excess information is critical.

Though many of us recognize the harmful effects of social media on our mental health, it can be hard to kick the habit—partly because it feels like we are connecting with others. But is that true? Is social media really providing us with positive social connections?

Interestingly, research shows otherwise. According to researchers,

> A study of nineteen- to thirty-two-year-olds revealed a strong linear association between increased social media usage and increased perceived social isolation. Researchers noted that one explanation for the results

may be that socially isolated individuals tend to spend more time on social media, while other studies have found that many online users aren't able to turn online interactions into "real" social relationships.[4]

We know the relationship between social media and social isolation is complex, and social isolation can't be entirely attributed to social media usage. But in 2019, the average person spent 144 minutes per day on social media, and a 2018 study found that "extensive social media usage is linked with decreased emotional wellness and lower satisfaction in interpersonal relationships."[5] In an article for The Gottman Institute, author Genesis Games offers a few simple tips for creating boundaries around social media. She notes that some of the best ways we can navigate the topic when it comes to those we love include things like prioritizing quality time without social media, checking in with loved ones or partners before we post about them, giving people the benefit of the doubt (as tone of voice is hard to gauge), and refusing to do or say anything online that you wouldn't do face-to-face.[6]

Part of our disconnect may be attributed to how we communicate with others: In a setting like social media, we use the screen as a mediator, missing out on some of the most essential factors in communicating well. One of these is nonverbal communication, which is integral to interacting with others.

Jacq Spence explains how our reliance on nonverbal communication plays out in the world around us:

> Every day, we communicate with our family, friends, colleagues, and even strangers, but only a small percentage of what we communicate during each of

these conversations is verbal. Research shows that the vast majority of what we convey through our interactions with others is innate and instinctual, known as nonverbal communication. Nonverbal behavior like body movements and posture, facial expressions, eye contact, hand gestures, and tone of voice all contribute to how we communicate and understand each other. Often, we are unaware of our participation in interpersonal, nonverbal communication because these actions are inherent to how we converse as humans and ingrained into our daily lives.[7]

In fact, Albert Mehrabian, who researches body language, found that when people are in face-to-face conversations, 55 percent of that communication is nonverbal, 38 percent is vocal, and only 7 percent are words alone.[8] It's no wonder we struggle to adapt to online communication.

Unfortunately, our online communication misses that crucial component.

In the article "Five Biblical Principles for Social Media," author Rob Brockman discusses how the Bible sheds important light on how Christians should speak to others in public—which, with the advent of social media, includes how we engage with people online.

Each time we decide to post online, there are five key questions to ask to measure the quality of our content:

1. Does the post stir up controversy or debate? (See Titus 3:1–2, 1 Timothy 2:8, and 2 Timothy 2:23.)

2. Is the post impulsive? Are we posting out of momentary frustration or irritation or after careful

thought and consideration? (See James 1:19–21, Titus 2:2–8, 1 Peter 4:7, and 2 Peter 1:5–8.)

3. Does the post demonstrate respect for all involved, marked by gentleness? (See 2 Timothy 2:23–25, 1 Timothy 4:12, Titus 3:2, and James 4:11.)

4. Does the topic fall under the category of gossip? [Just because it is true does not mean it is helpful or necessary to say!] (See Proverbs 20:19, 2 Timothy 2:16, 1 Timothy 4:7, James 1:26, and Matthew 12:36.)

5. Is the goal of the posting to glorify Him and spread His message or to garner attention for ourselves? (See Ephesians 4:29, 1 Thessalonians 5:11, and Romans 14:19.)[9]

It can be tempting to use social media to fulfill our need for affirmation or attention or simply because we're bored. When we fall into those categories, it may be time to step away from social media and open up the Word. As the author concludes, "In 2 Corinthians 5, Paul will tell us that out of fear of God (vs. 11), we seek to persuade others out of love (vs. 14), to be reconciled to God (vs. 19), as ambassadors of Christ to this world (vs. 20), with a ministry of reconciliation! There is nothing that social media can give you that is better than Gospel purpose!"[10]

Although social media can help us keep in touch with those we might otherwise not see regularly, spending time together in person is necessary for our social and emotional well-being. Dan Buettner is an author who often writes on longevity and happiness and has focused some of his work on the "Blue Zones," which are geographic areas in the world where people experience low rates of chronic disease and tend to live longer. Buettner discusses nine components of maintaining a long, healthy life with vitality in his book *The Blue Zones Solution: Eating and Living Like the World's Healthiest People*. Interestingly, three lessons he's learned from the world's longest-living people involve connecting with others.

The first is to nurture your spirit by finding a faith community. According to Buettner, "Most centenarians that researchers talked to belonged to a faith-based community. Practicing meditation or yoga is another way to shut down mind chatter and get in touch with your spiritual side."[11] Second, the author notes that leaning on loved ones is essential. "Close family ties across generations leads to children, grandchildren, and extended family honoring and supporting adults throughout their lives."[12] Third—and as we've noted, just as importantly—we must build strong social networks. As the article says, "Keep old friends and make new ones. Participating regularly in social activities protects against the harmful physical and emotional consequences of social isolation."[13]

Of course, our online connections can be beneficial in certain situations. I recently spoke to a therapist about increased telehealth visits for mental well-being since the COVID-19 pandemic. She acknowledged the benefit of easing access. However, she said face-to-face is often necessary, especially around trauma or challenging personal issues. Our in-person relationships give us clearer, more intimate, believable, and palpable connections.

Strategies to Reconnect—With Ourselves and Others

One message I've heard from women is that they yearn for a simpler, more connected life. A law student in her twenties told me how she had worked to shift her attention:

Social media is training us to compare our lives instead
of appreciating everything that we are! I often wonder
how simple and carefree life was before the internet
made it so easy for others to comment on our lives.
I [have] stopped worrying about taking the "perfect"
pictures to post on social media and begun to enjoy
life and all of the beauty it has to offer.

A registered dietician in her late forties echoed this idea:
"The more I've grown in Christ and the less time I spend on
media, I find myself not bombarded with thoughts of insecurity
about beauty."

Comparison can often fuel envy, and a lack of contentment
with our lives can cause additional stress. Although it's essential
to have strong social relationships, it's equally important to
recognize how we can foster contentment and less stress in our
own lives.

After all, stress is destroying our physical and mental
health. Up to 75 percent of primary care visits include mental
or behavioral health components.[14] The body doesn't know or
care what caused the stress; it simply knows it is experiencing
it. One of the ways this shows up in the body is through the
stress hormones adrenaline and cortisol. According to the Mayo
Clinic, these play an important role in the body:

Adrenaline increases your heart rate, elevates your
blood pressure, and boosts energy supplies. Cortisol,
the primary stress hormone, increases sugars (glucose)
in the bloodstream, enhances your brain's use of glucose, and increases the availability of substances that
repair tissues. Cortisol also curbs functions that would

be nonessential or harmful in a fight-or-flight situation. It alters immune system responses and suppresses the digestive system, the reproductive system, and growth processes. This complex natural alarm system also communicates with the brain regions that control mood, motivation, and fear.[15]

Once the perceived threat passes, the hormone levels should return to normal. But in our fast-paced culture, our fight-or-flight reaction remains activated all too often. Over time, this long-term exposure to elevated cortisol and other stress hormones increases our risk of health problems, including anxiety, depression, digestive issues, headaches, muscle tension and pain, heart problems (including heart disease, heart attack, high blood pressure, and stroke), sleep problems, weight gain, and impaired memory and concentration.[16]

One important technique we can use to offset the stress of the world is mindfulness. We can use mindfulness to quiet our minds and spirits. Being mindful is not mysticism or a religious exercise; it is a calming practice and way of life.

Mindfulness is paying attention. It is noticing what you are doing, feeling, and thinking at the time you are doing, feeling, and thinking it.

As Boyd Bailey notes, "Stillness sets you free from busyness that can betray your trust in God."[17] Mindfulness is challenging in our age of distraction. Many of us live complicated, overly busy lives crammed with work or looking for a job, caring for children or aging parents, school, volunteering, commuting, health issues, and money worries.

Paying attention requires both effort and trust. The effort comes in choosing to "set your mind on things above" (Col. 3:2) and "renew your mind" (Rom. 12:2). In fact, that entire verse is instructive: "Do not conform to the pattern of this world, but be transformed by the renewing of your mind. Then you will be able to test and approve what God's will is—his good, pleasing and perfect will" (Rom. 12:2).

Once you recognize that the pattern of this world is to multitask, want more, and regret what is lost, it's easy to see how mindfulness exemplifies what it means to renew your mind.

So, what are some steps to help us be mindful, breathe, and find mental peace?

First, start by focusing on who is in control. Memorize scripture to help refocus your thoughts. Here are a few to get you started:

✞ Test me, Lord, and try me, examine my heart and my mind; for I have always been mindful of your unfailing love and have lived in reliance on your faithfulness. (Ps. 26:2–3)

✞ Cease striving and know that I am God; I will be exalted among the nations, I will be exalted in the earth. (Ps. 46:10 NASB 1995)

✞ Know that the Lord Himself is God; It is He who has made us, and not we ourselves; We are His people and the sheep of His pasture. (Ps. 100:3)

A simple way to help "fix your thoughts on Jesus" (Heb. 3:1) is to set an alarm on your watch, cellphone, or computer to think about God. When it rings, take that moment to "set your mind on things above" (Col. 3:2). Do this several times each day.

Along with refocusing on God, you can take steps to shut out the noise. It's okay to have boundaries that limit the chaos of this world. Remember, as Anne Lamott says, "'No' is a complete sentence."[18] People love to talk about everything wrong in this world, but listening to a constant stream of negativity from 24-hour news and our social media channels is paralyzing. Choose to limit or stop the noise altogether.

Several recent studies revealed that even one month off of Facebook and other social media resulted in improved overall health and well-being.[19] Even Sean Parker, the former president of Facebook, has said that the platform was designed to give you a dopamine hit with social validation that makes you addicted and leads to distraction.[20]

Like social media, though our cell phones are helpful, they provide easy access to information and entertainment. They can create distractions that compete with children and other drivers for our attention. Even when we are face-to-face with others, our minds may be so filled with checklists that the person in front of us disappears, as does the moment we are supposed to share with them. The average smartphone user touches their phone 2,617 times a day.[21] So, take a break and limit yourself! You will be happier.

Moving Forward

There's a Fourth of July gathering that, years later, still lingers in my mind. At the time, I was in my residency after medical school. Most of my extended family had congregated at my parents' home, and cousins, aunts, and uncles gathered around the tables, eating, laughing, and catching up. We lived all over the country, so there typically were four to five conversations at any given time. I loved it. I always loved being with family, playing games, and listening to stories.

On this particular occasion, however, I was distracted. I was anxious about a large presentation due the following week and felt torn between continuing the conversation or going to my room to work on my presentation. Finally, I decided that I should leave. As I excused myself, one of my cousins said, "You just don't want to be around us because we are not doctors. You have had it so easy in life and just had this MD degree handed to you because your father is a doctor."

I was stunned. I felt hurt by the accusation but even more so by the suggestion that a family member could so easily discount my hard work and character. Of course, there have been many times when I felt misunderstood by friends or family members. That happens to all of us due to ineffective communication, lack of communication, or disinterest. Yet the ability to ignore the desire to compare ourselves with others requires us to know and love ourselves first and foremost.

So how do we balance our desire to be known in this world without falling prey to becoming a chameleon that changes based on our circumstances? How do we stay true to who we are, show up authentically, and allow others to do the same without harmful comparisons that make us feel like we are competing? How do we learn to explore who we are in Christ and then bring our whole selves to our relationships, conversations, and encounters in a way that embraces humanity?

Our country has stooped to a place of continual bullying and division, pitting people against people based on everything from political policy to hair color. We can and must decide to treat all people with respect, kindness, and love. Only then can we begin discussions from a place of integrity and safety, creating a foundation for us to call each other to higher ground and grow in understanding and kindness. It's only then that social media and other forms of communication allow us to make this world a better and kinder place.

Each of us is a masterpiece of the High and Holy King, and we are lovely. We are known and adored by Him! When we find our worth in Him, other comparisons fade and are less challenging. Comparisons only hold us back and lead to jealousy, envy, gossip, and covetousness. As President Theodore Roosevelt reportedly said, "Comparison is the thief of joy."

Yet refusing to compare ourselves with one another is easier said than done. After all, comparisons begin early in life but can be exacerbated by social media as we age. It's no wonder that teenage depression, addiction, and suicide are at an all-time high or that bullying, fear, and anger are pervasive problems in our country. Even if we survive the teen and college years with our hearts and self-worth intact, plenty of comparisons lead to guilt or shame. If we're single, we notice images of perfect couples who are in love and married. Whether we have children or not, stay at home or work outside the home, homeschool or have our children in a public or private school, or make organic baby food or breastfeed—in all areas of life, we are inundated with "helpful" information and opinions.

Let's remove ourselves from the endless round of comparison. Instead, let's make our own decisions prayerfully. Allow and trust other women to do the same. Then, find a few women who are safe, loyal, and honest confidants to help you gain an outside perspective.

Lord willing, we are all on a path of growth and maturity in our faith, experiences, and choices. As we allow others to know us and lean in to know others, let us do so through a lens of kindness and understanding. Let us be women who can thoughtfully hold others' words, affirmations, and thoughts in a place of listening, not comparison, which can lead to division.

What changes can we make today to show up differently and engage in our relationships in a life-giving way? First, let's start by resolving to recognize and truly see people for who they are in their authentic, non-social-media lives.

My husband and I were walking by a small playground recently full of several young children playing on the playground slides, swings, and a seesaw. One little boy was standing on the top of the slide, ready to slide down. I am sure for his small size, tackling this slide required courage, and he desired that others see him accomplish this feat. He stood there for several moments, yelling at a little girl named Jane.

"Jane, see ME! Jane—hey, Jane—SEE ME! JAAANNE, SEEEEEE MEEEE!"

Jane was busy playing with something else and never once looked up.

Watching him broke my heart, and I found myself chiming in, "Jane! Hey, *Jane*!! Your friend wants you to look at him on the slide. Please, *look*!"

Finally, the little boy shrugged his shoulders, slid down the slide, then went to sit and watch others. His great brave move was left unseen by Jane.

Although you and I don't need anyone to cheer us on the playground, isn't it true that we all have the innate desire to be seen and known by others? We all want others to witness our courageous moments and overlook our not-so-brave moments. Each of us is created in the *Imago Dei*—the image of God—and worthy of being seen and appreciated for who we are. Let's begin by noticing those around us in all their uniqueness and complexity away from the distortion of social media.

When we do, we'll be better equipped to serve others—and, by extension, God's Kingdom. When we can truly see the people that God puts in our path, we'll be able to embrace the opportunity to serve and mentor others along their way and in their faith.

One of the best ways to notice others around us is to recognize our own value—we, too, are created in the image of God! Remember that God is always with you and sees you even when you feel unseen. Start your days with affirmative thoughts that solidify God's truths about you and define your worth. This practice will help you enter the world with confidence and curiosity as you meet and interact with others, either in person or online. And when conversations become the type that slight the worth of you or others, be the voice of redirection and do not accept that rhetoric. You may lose some friendships, but the ones you maintain will be fulfilling and authentic.

Although we live in this world, it's not our home. It's a world that, by its very nature, forces us to think of ourselves and our immediate wants, needs, and desires. This world can often pit our selfish human nature against our God-given call to serve others. When we ask God to guide us, we can embrace technology's advances without wandering off course from His higher goals and good. Although we should not be afraid to use technology and social media, we must be ever mindful that we desire to please God in how we use it. Ask God to show you the people He would ask you to see every day—those whom you can serve and mentor to help them see who Jesus desires to be in their life.

After all, we need each other. We thrive most when we are in relationships that will not only empower us but stretch us to grow to our fullest potential.

S N A P

Seek Him

As you focus on being proactive about your social connections and behavior, whether in person or online, choose to measure motives and messaging by His Word.

MEDITATE ON THESE WORDS

☩ It is for freedom that Christ has set us free. Stand firm, then, and do not let yourselves be burdened again by a yoke of slavery. (Gal. 5:1 NIV)

☩ Test me, Lord, and try me, examine my heart and my mind; for I have always been mindful of your unfailing love and have lived in reliance on your faithfulness. (Ps. 26:2–3)

☩ He says, "Be still, and know that I am God; I will be exalted among the nations, I will be exalted in the earth." (Ps. 46:10)

☩ Know that the LORD Himself is God; It is He who has made us, and not we ourselves; We are his people and the sheep of His pasture. (Ps. 100:3 NASB 1995)

✞ Set your minds on things above, not on earthly things. (Col. 3:2 NIV)

✞ Therefore, holy brothers and sisters, who share in the heavenly calling, fix your thoughts on Jesus, whom we acknowledge as our apostle and high priest. (Heb. 3:1)

Nourish Self

Mindfulness is being mindful and aware of what you are doing and thinking as you do or think about it. Developing a consistent mindfulness practice is vital to gaining and maintaining a healthy social connection, whether in person or on social media.

Some apps help guide you in a mindfulness practice that you can download on your phone. Some ask you to be seated and quiet with your eyes closed. Others can be used while walking or driving. You can typically choose the length of the mindfulness practice for each session, from a few minutes to an hour.

This mindfulness practice is often centered around our breathing because our breath is always with us, even though we are not always aware of it.

Activity 1: Try a deep breathing exercise.

Get a handheld mirror out and practice breathing in through your nose for a count of four, holding it for a count of four, and then breathing out through your mouth with enough force to fog up your mirror.

Do this three times in a row, several times during the day, to ease stress and gain awareness.

Activity 2: Journal your thoughts.

When we journal statements about ourselves that are positive and true, we can relieve anxiety, loneliness, and depression.

Consider this question: *What thoughts in my head are robbing me of my peace?* Write them down, and then pray for ways to surrender those. Ask God if there is anything that you can do to alleviate the feelings, and then trust His faithfulness.

Write down three names of people you would like to reach out to that day:

- Someone you know well whom you would like to speak to about an issue or problem you are facing to ask for wisdom or insight.

- Someone who may be lonely and could benefit from you checking in on how they are doing or what they need.

- Someone you barely know but would like to know better to explore a way to connect.

Survey your response whenever you feel the urge to check in with your social media sites. Note which posts make you feel worse about yourself, monopolize your time, and keep you from being present in real life.

Before you post online, pause, and go through a mental exercise to ask yourself why you want to post. Do not post if it is simply to be noticed or affirmed. Instead, pause and remember you do not need affirmation from anyone to feel worthy or valuable.

Activity 3: Rethink your bedtime habits.

Resting well restores our peace and makes it easier to rest in His truths instead of seeking approval from others.

Here are a few more tips for a great night of sleep:

- Limit your bedroom to sleep rather than working or doing other things in the space. This signals to your body that entering this room begins the go-to-sleep process of unwinding and relaxing.

- Go to bed and get up at approximately the same time each day. Doing so conditions your internal clock.

- Keep your bedroom uncluttered and dark.

- Unplug the phone and use earplugs if the street is noisy.

- Do not drink beverages with caffeine or consume chocolate, spicy foods, fatty foods, and medication with stimulants before bed.

- Keep your bedroom at a comfortable temperature (70° F).

- Don't exercise within two hours of bedtime.

- Select a comfortable pillow and mattress.

Activity 4: Go through your social media posts from the past six months and ask God to reveal the motivation behind each one.

Was it to gain attention, followers, prestige, social connection, or new friends? Or was it a resource or tool to help you and others on their faith journey?

Moving forward, pause before posting on social media and measure the content by God's Word. Then delete or unfollow anything or anyone that does not bring you joy and freedom in Christ.

Activity 5: Every week, intentionally plan to reach out to someone that you do not normally get to see but would like to spend some time with and schedule a connection.

That could be a phone call, FaceTime, coffee, lunch, walk, or other activity. This does not have to take much time, but consider expanding this invitation to someone outside of your normal friend group (or it can be someone you know fairly well that you can know better). This could also include volunteering somewhere in your community. Serving others brings incredible connection.

Activity 6: Set device-free times daily to foster peace of mind and productivity.

Doing so will also improve your personal relationship skills.

Armor of God

Pretend you are placing a helmet on your head. Doing so reminds me of the first time our daughter had her unrestricted license and was going to drive herself and her two younger brothers to school. She was all set, waiting for them one morning, when our middle son walked into the room wearing his bike helmet and knee and elbow pads. Despite our chuckles, my daughter did not find our son's attempt to equip himself for safety on the "perilous" ride to school humorous. But even though my son didn't need the helmet that day, the point is that a helmet is protective in nature.

In the same way, the helmet of salvation helps to guard our minds from external forces. Consider making that gesture today—settling a helmet on your head—in the morning. When you do, the visual reminder will help you set your mind on God's Kingdom throughout the day. Think of genuinely seeing each person in front of you with a desire to show them Jesus.

Prayer

DEAR LORD,

AM SO GRATEFUL FOR MY RELATIONSHIP WITH YOU, above all others. May I be reminded daily of the influence I can have on others with my in-person and online connections and relationships. Help me to be thoughtful and let my light shine for all to see You in me.

Put Your protective shield around all my relationships. Guide me in guarding my thoughts, actions, and words to others so that You alone are honored and glorified. Help me to remove any unhealthy or unholy aspects of my communication.

In His name,

Amen.

CHAPTER 6

Sticks and Stones
May Break My Bones,
But Words Can Crush My Spirit

*T*HERE IS SOMETHING EXTRAORDINARY ABOUT A HOT CUP of tea. As a teenager, my mother and I would sit in our two favorite chairs in our den and sip hot tea before school or the start of the day. We "solved" many problems. But mostly, we paused long enough to get to know each other and share some of our inner thoughts. It was a treasured time that made memories and forged bonds.

During medical school, I followed the crowd of coffee drinkers and had my share of coffee intake to fuel a sleep-deprived body. However, I eventually returned to my love of tea for its taste and health benefits.

My daughter Rebecca was intrigued by my love of tea early on. She would recruit her two younger brothers as guests at our afternoon tea parties on the couch or porch with our Disney Mrs. Potts Teapot and Chip Teacups. We chatted about friends, toys, fashion, and life as we held our pinkies up, sipping lemonade or raspberry tea. We giggled like little girls while the boys tolerated us. I told them they were preparing to be great listeners for future relationships.

Even though Rebecca and I have continued to admire and anticipate our hot tea, the real enjoyment is the communication we share.

There have been so many books written about the importance of communication. Yet, in our technologically advanced
culture, the art of face-to-face talking and listening is dimin-
ishing, which is tragic. Open and honest communication can
make us feel vulnerable and is often difficult. However, there
is no substitute for talking. Our most open communication
should be shared with the few "safe" people in our lives.

Words can help or harm. Yet, as Christians, we are called
to season our words with grace. When we spend time with
God, we cultivate our ability to assume the best by considering
others and their intentions. This generous mindset can only
occur when we develop a settled mind that defines our value
based on who God says we are, leading to a mental toughness
that is impervious to others' negative opinions. Once developed,
this mindset can overcome our greatest critic: our inner voice.
Words hold incredible power! Words spoken aloud influence
how we think about ourselves. We can speak positive affirmations that embolden, encourage, and empower us. Think of
saying to yourself out loud: *I am worthy! I am important! I am
bold! I am beautiful! I am loved! I've got this!*

The Original Communicator

God is our best example of healthy communication. We glean
life-giving concepts by examining how God has communicated
with His people over the years. During the Patriarchal Age, God
spoke directly to the leading patriarchs—or fathers—about
what they were to do. Their role was to be still, listen to Him,
and heed His instructions. As the biblical community moved
from the Patriarchal Age to the Mosaic Age and then to the
Christian Age, God changed His method of communication.

Although God has spoken through people, angels, a burning bush, a cloud, and the wind, the most accurate picture of who God is and how He sees us is embodied in Jesus. Studying the Word of God—including the words Jesus spoke during His ministry on earth—is integral to understanding God and how He has chosen to communicate with us. As the Bible reminds us, in the "last days He has spoken in His Son" (Heb. 1:2) and the Word. Hebrews 4:12 (ESV) is clear on the power of the Word in growing our faith: "For the word of God is living and active, sharper than any two-edged sword, piercing to the division of soul and of spirit, of joints and of marrow, and discerning the thoughts and intentions of the heart."

Yet no matter how He communicates, He is everywhere, all the time. As Paul writes in Colossians 1:17, "He is before all things, and in Him all things hold together" (NASB 1995). As we seek to hear Him, our role is to take the posture of Romans 10:17, reading God's Word and bolstering our faith: "So faith comes from hearing, and hearing through the word of Christ." When we spend time in God's Word—reading, meditating, and memorizing it—then we will follow Him. As John 10:27 reminds us, this process is vital to deepening our relationship with Jesus, "My sheep hear My voice, and I know them, and they follow Me."

Ladies, we are relational by nature. We love and crave deep, meaningful relationships, which only happen from spending time with people. We lean in, listen, learn, and love. The same is true for developing a deeper relationship with our Lord. Spending time in His Word and in prayer trains our ears, minds, and hearts to know Him. This type of active listening is vital to healthy communication.

As a teenager, I often approached my grandmother for advice. Still, I remember one time when I asked her advice about something I considered very important. She asked me why I came to her for guidance and direction. I told her she had a unique perspective on what was truly important. She would say, "Mary Evelyn, pretend as if you are eighty and looking back on this decision. What would you do? What would seem to be the wisest decision? What action would you wish you had taken? Your perspective on life is much more clear toward the end of life. Think like this, and you will know what to do."

Her profound words taught me lessons in wisdom and discernment for life's decisions. She knew that I understood and encouraged me constantly to make decisions with the end of my life in mind. I have never forgotten that. The Lord reminds us to keep this long-term perspective throughout scripture, especially in Psalms and Proverbs.

Let's be women who are slow and thoughtful with our words and decisions. Let's be women who seek God in the pursuit of that wisdom. Start by communicating your concerns to God, family, and trusted friends, praying and listening to what others and God say. He does not always answer audibly, but He hears and responds. As James says, "If any of you lacks wisdom, let him ask God, who gives generously to all without reproach, and it will be given him" (James 1:5 ESV).

Technology and Our Families

Several years ago, an episode of *The Oprah Show* focused on families. As an experiment, the show asked several families to give up technology, dining out, and a fast-paced lifestyle for seven days and spend quality family time together. The *Oprah* crew went to their homes and removed their computers, television sets, phones, computer and video games, and all other technological equipment. They then filmed the families over the following week.

At first, the families were in culture shock. They were miserable and didn't want to talk to their family members. They didn't want to go to the grocery store together to decide what to fix for dinner. One young teenager even said, "Oh, no. I can't eat vegetables. I am allergic to them." The thought of sitting down to eat dinner together was foreign.

After about three days, however, they were pleasantly surprised by what they learned about each other at the dinner table. They enjoyed the conversation and commented on how much fun it was.

They eagerly awaited the *Oprah* crew to return their items after seven days. Instead, the representative gave them one more option: They could have their things back or go seven more days without them. The family's mother was the only one who voted to get the items returned that day. She missed her cell phone and television shows. Overall, the experience changed the family for good.[1]

The technological era we live in has so many incredible advantages; however, we must intentionally maintain communication with one another. We can utilize and enjoy technology while still valuing face-to-face conversation. We know this to be true, but for some reason, we allow this world's urgent, enticing, fast-paced distractions to consume us. By keeping computers and televisions in family gathering places to be used together, we can minimize technology's prominence in our day-to-day lives. By placing boundaries on our phones and creating time when phones are in a shared basket or other holding place to minimize the temptation to look at them continually, we must live in the moment and be more fully present.

Even when we take the time to communicate with others, we sometimes can be very ineffective. When my husband Shawn and I were engaged, he was doing a general surgery internship in Buffalo, New York, and I was in my sophomore year of medical school in Louisville, Kentucky. Our communication could have been better, but we tried. Our engagement was before the day of cell phones, and with his busy schedule, we would grab a phone call on a landline whenever possible.

After spending a week in my hometown of Paducah, Kentucky, picking out china, crystal, and silverware, I wanted Shawn's input. So I called him in Buffalo when I knew he would be available and gave him the list of choices, asking him to try to get to a store and see if he approved of what I'd picked out. He wanted to let me know he was engaged in the decision-making, so when he called me after visiting the store, he suggested one change to the informal dinnerware: Iris on Grey instead of Poppies on Blue. I definitely wanted Poppies on Blue, but I honored his wish since it was the only thing he mentioned.

Years later—probably twelve to fifteen years after we wed—in the heat of an argument, I told him that I had always wished we had picked the Poppies on Blue.

He couldn't believe that it really mattered to me. He said the choice had not been that important to him, but he wanted me to know that he was interested enough to visit the store and review the options. Although we had spoken to each other, we failed to communicate because of our efforts to please one another.

During this same demanding year, I repeatedly reminded Shawn to ask his potential groomsmen if they would like to be part of the wedding so I could communicate details to them. After several weeks, he told me he had asked all of them, so I sent out my detailed information letter. A week later, one of them stopped me at the hospital while we were both working and asked if the letter meant he was *in* the wedding. Confused, I wondered whether Shawn had asked him to be a groomsman earlier. He said, "Well, Shawn called me and said you were getting married and to 'Be there, dude.'" Hmm. Was that communicating? To Shawn, it was, yet to his friend, the message was unclear. We have laughed about this many times and marveled at how we can assume we are communicating clearly when we are not.

Words can also be contagious, especially when it comes to their energy. For instance, when I started my medical practice thirty years ago, I had a lot to learn about the business aspects of running a dermatology office, especially personnel management. Often, an employee would approach me with a huffy tone of voice and say, "Dr. Evelyn, you are going to be so mad . . ." Taking my cue from their energy, I would feel upset before knowing the issue. Over time, Proverbs 18:13 (NLT) provided the wisdom I needed to remind me to pause: "Spouting off before listening to the facts is both shameful and foolish." I had to learn to separate their delivery from the message and not take on their personal feelings as my own.

Our words, the energy behind the words, and nonverbal cues are powerful communicators. We are swayed quite easily by the combination of these three things, and I have regretted many times when I spoke or reacted too quickly. It has taken me years and experience to separate the overall message from the energy and feelings of the person uttering the words. Yet doing so is one aspect of stewarding communication.

Communication combines listening, pondering (using discernment), and speaking. All aspects are critical for us to be effective and godly in our speech and nonverbal communication.

When our children were small, we strived to have them use three simple, easy-to-remember words before speaking: Stop, look, and listen.

When you feel you must say something and are bursting from the seams, take a breath and stop, look, and listen.

- **Stop:** Stop speaking, stop running into the room, and stop the angst in your spirit.

- **Look:** Look around the room, look into the person's eyes in front of you, and look into your own heart for the purpose behind your message that makes it feel necessary to deliver.

- **Listen:** Listen to who is speaking and what is being said, be curious, and lean in to truly listen—devoid of any ego or desire to express your words first, as beautiful and paramount as they may be.

Once you have done these three things, then your words will most likely be "seasoned with grace" and received as your heart intends. Or, as Proverbs 18:20 reminds us, "Wise words satisfy like a good meal; the right words bring satisfaction."

In Joshua Becker's podcast *Becoming Minimalist*, he discusses how, in our journey to declutter, what we really must do is "de-own."[2] In Emily Freeman's book *The Next Right Thing*, she applies this concept to the soul. The wounds of this life, day-to-day interactions, and frustrations stick to us deep in our souls. To truly walk this life in freedom from that heaviness, we need to find a way to not only declutter our soul but to de-own those thorns we carry.[3] The Lord guides us to "Be still and know that I am God" in Psalm 46:10. Spending time in silence, mindfully listening to God as I quiet my mind and body, is a reset. Sometimes, it is as simple as walking into another room to take four deep breaths in and out. Other times, we cannot remove ourselves from an interaction. Still, we can settle our spirit simply by recounting a scripture, becoming aware of our breathing, or stopping to listen and refusing to own the emotions around us.

I do not know what strategies will be most helpful to you, but we must each take the time to de-own those hurtful remnants in our souls, minds, and hearts. Are you carrying around some unkind words someone spoke to you years ago or even yesterday? Do you regret kind deeds left undone or unkind acts that harmed a loved one? Have you not been able to shake the burden of gaining comfort from unhealthy choices? Is it difficult to accept the consequences of past mistakes and move on?

The messages we speak and receive throughout our days matter. When someone called me fat, skinny, or silly as a child, it hurt to the core. Years later, I still remember the words that were spoken and the person who said them.

Most of us regret things we've said or done. But God has not called us to live in the past but to look ahead to His greater purpose. We gain freedom and peace as we choose to forgive ourselves and others. As C. S. Lewis said, "Every time you make a choice, you are turning the central part of you, the part that chooses, into something a little different from what it was before."[4] By stewarding our lives in a way that continually looks to God's words and believes them to our core, we become more fully alive and complete in Him.

However, sometimes the best thing to do is to stay silent, which may be the most difficult. Sometimes, we can extend grace, mercy, and love to another who has just wounded us, accepting that they are on their own journey and not ready to advance. Sometimes, the right thing is to say and do nothing and trust God.

Communicating With Ourselves

While communicating with others—and healing internal wounds from past interactions—is important, many of us struggle to find ways to communicate with ourselves in helpful ways.

As a woman in her early forties who had just gone through a divorce told me,

> I find I am my own worst enemy. I am the one who keeps myself from healing. I do not feel like I am good enough and am a constant work in progress. I want to see my true beauty, but the constant in-your-face images of what society thinks you should look, feel, or be like is very hard. I also struggle with words that have been spoken to me that make me feel less than others. My own thoughts keep me from my best life. When someone speaks negatively to me, that is what I tend to believe about myself.

Living a life of kindness and intention is hard if we constantly criticize ourselves. So how can we begin cultivating a life that recognizes our beauty and self-worth? Most of us struggle with being our own worst bully. The Bible provides some important clues to help get us started. Proverbs 17:22 (AMPC) says, "A happy heart is good medicine and a cheerful mind works healing . . ." God desires for us to make time for fun and enjoy our life. There is beauty in playfulness, fun, and joy in a person.

It's important to understand what joy is. It's not about entertaining yourself, getting your way all the time, or laughing constantly. Joy can be expressed as extreme hilarity, calm delight, and everything in between! It can be something I like to call "little happies." My whole body feels better when I chuckle at a funny joke, observe someone who is okay with laughing at themselves, get a prime parking spot that lets me pull through to the other side, watch the sunset, play a card game with dear friends (and celebrate whoever wins), obtain a personal record when lifting weights with my trainer, learn something new about my profession, delight in deep reflection on a fresh perspective to a Bible verse, or taste a new recipe.

In fact, Nehemiah 8:10 says the joy of the Lord is our strength. And we need that strength every day. As Don Colbert notes, "Joy does not flow from situations. It flows from your will and your emotions deep within. You can choose to be joyful, or you can choose to be miserable. Nobody can make these inner choices for you."[5]

Looking to boost your joy? Try these ideas:

- Smile. Your day will go as the corners of your mouth turn. Smile at other people, too—smiling is nearly a universal language.

- Lighten up. I know life can be so heavy that it feels hard to breathe, but make yourself smile. So many studies on laughter and health show that our health is directly linked to something as simple as a smile, chuckle, or belly laugh.

- Be happy and thank God daily because He created you for a purpose. Laugh, have fun, and remember to enjoy life. Learn to cherish the small things. Count your blessings daily.

So many people have the mindset that they will be happy and enjoy life when something specific happens—when they go on vacation, when the kids are older, when they get higher on the ladder of success at work, when they get married—the list could go on and on.

I want you to get this important truth: God wants you to enjoy your life *now*, not *when*. As someone once said, "Enjoy the little things in life, for one day you'll look back and realize they were big things" (Anonymous).

One of the most practical ways to increase our joy is through laughter. As Don Colbert reminds us,

> Laughter is good medicine. Loma Linda University Medical Center's Dr. Lee Berk has studied the healing benefits of laughter. He concluded that laughter boosts the immune system and reduces dangerous stress hormones in the body. In one study involving sixteen men who watched a funny video, levels of the stress hormone cortisol fell 39 percent after a good belly laugh. Adrenaline levels fell 70 percent, while levels of the feel-good hormone endorphin rose 27 percent. And growth hormone (the youth hormone) levels skyrocketed 87 percent.[6]

Those statistics are staggering! Colbert also notes that "the average adult laughs twenty-five times a day and the average child four hundred times a day."[7] So, as Jesus said, let's be like these little children. They can help show us the way to relearn joy.

Along with laughter, we can learn another lesson from children by developing a sense of play. When we choose to be creative in our play—through painting, dancing, bubbles and polka dots, cooking, photography, and calligraphy—our spirits will lighten.

When my sweet mom was in the middle stages of dementia, I would stop in and see her regularly. One week, I kept noticing more and more yellow sticky notes appearing on the walls, counters, bookcases, television, and microwave. A sweet smile formed when I got close enough to read them. In her desire to hold onto joy in a challenging season, she had written this Bible verse on sticky notes and placed them everywhere: "A cheerful heart is good medicine" (Prov. 17:22 NIV).

Reframing Our Experiences through Gratitude

I took my daughter to New York for her birthday a few years ago. We planned to visit museums, see a Broadway play or musical, eat at good restaurants, and walk in Central Park. She was in college at the time and called me two days before meeting in New York, excited to tell me that she had signed us up for a yoga workshop!

Now, I love yoga and understand the benefits of it; however, I enjoy my level of yoga. My daughter is a yoga instructor and is much more advanced.

So I paused and asked, "Hmm, what type of yoga workshop, dear?"

She replied, "Oh, it is a four-hour intensive yoga and writing workshop with a visiting yoga instructor I have always wanted to take a class with."

To say I was a little nervous the day we took the subway to the area in New York City where the workshop would take place is an understatement. I did not want to hold my daughter back or take away from her experience; however, I could see myself passing out on the mat two hours into the workshop.

I not only survived, I *enjoyed* it. The class was filled with moments of intense yoga work and sweating, followed by pauses to write to a prompt the instructor provided.

Science shows that when we work out intensely, our thoughts flow more freely, and we can write with less structure and less self-critiquing. Yet the most memorable part was a new practice that my daughter and I began after the instructor suggested it. She asked us to consider finding an accountability partner to send three to five beautiful things we were grateful for to each other in a daily text message. The items did not need to be big things, but noting them fostered a daily awareness of gratitude.

We started doing that with each other at least a few mornings a week for several years, and we loved it. Though the exercise can seem contrived, it still boosts our awareness and perspective.

Reframing our identity through gratitude is one of the best ways to reconsider other things that affect our well-being, including how we see ourselves. As noted earlier in the chapter, how we talk to ourselves influences other parts of our lives, including how we define our purpose. A fitness trainer and massage therapist in her mid-forties got to the heart of this challenge when she told me how her inner thought life played out:

> I think my negative thoughts and attitudes are the
> biggest stumbling blocks to me living out my life

of true beauty and freedom. Allowing my negative emotions to have power creates an inner atmosphere that is not conducive to the flow of beauty. Seeing stress as negative instead of a powerful motivator thwarts growth. What is the magic between service and peace? How is it that by lifting others, I am the one who is blessed? And isn't that when I am the most beautiful? When the image of Christ in me is reflected for others to see?

When we redefine the inner landscape of our lives through joy, play, and gratitude and see the beauty of ourselves in our God-given identity, we can move forward with purposeful joy into reclaiming our lives, using them for His glory. As we do, we'll be better equipped to communicate the message of God's love to the world.

S N A P

Seek Him

Meditate on God's words as you hone your inner and outer dialogue. Place these verses somewhere that encourages you to memorize them. Then your words will be seasoned with His grace in your daily conversations.

MEDITATE ON THESE WORDS

✝ And now in these final days, he has spoken to us through his Son. God promised everything to the Son as an inheritance, and through the Son he created the universe. (Heb. 1:2 NLT)

✝ For the word of God is alive and powerful. It is sharper than the sharpest two-edged sword, cutting between soul and spirit, between joint and marrow. It exposes our innermost thoughts and desires. (Heb. 4:12)

✝ He existed before anything else, and he holds all creation together. (Col. 1:17)

✝ So faith comes from hearing, that is, hearing the Good News about Christ. (Rom. 10:17)

✝ My sheep listen to my voice; I know them, and they follow me. (John 10:27)

✝ Spouting off before listening to the facts is both shameful and foolish. (Prov. 18:13)

✝ Wise words satisfy like a good meal; the right words bring satisfaction. (Prov. 18:20)

✝ Be still, and know that I am God! I will be honored by every nation. I will be honored throughout the world. (Ps. 46:10)

✝ A cheerful heart is good medicine, but a broken spirit saps a person's strength. (Prov. 17:22)

✝ And Nehemiah continued, "Go and celebrate with a feast of rich foods and sweet drinks, and share gifts of food with people who have nothing prepared. This is a sacred day before our Lord. Don't be dejected and sad, for the joy of the LORD is your strength!" (Neh. 8:10)

✝ Don't worry about anything; instead, pray about everything. Tell God what you need, and thank him for all he has done. Then you will experience God's peace, which exceeds anything we can understand. His peace will guard your hearts and minds as you live in Christ Jesus.

And now, dear brothers and sisters, one final thing. Fix your thoughts on what is true, and honorable, and right, and pure, and lovely, and admirable. Think about things that are excellent and worthy of praise. (Phil. 4:6–8)

✝ That is why I tell you not to worry about everyday life—whether you have enough food and drink, or enough clothes to wear. Isn't life more than food, and your body more than clothing? Look at the birds. They don't plant or harvest or store food in barns, for your heavenly Father feeds them. And aren't you far more valuable to him than they are? Can all your worries add a single moment to your life?

And why worry about your clothing? Look at the lilies of the field and how they grow. They don't work or make their clothing, yet Solomon in all his glory was not dressed as beautifully as they are. And if God cares so wonderfully for wildflowers that are here today and thrown into the fire tomorrow, he will certainly care for you. Why do you have so little faith?

So don't worry about these things, saying, "What will we eat? What will we drink? What will we wear?" These things dominate the thoughts of unbelievers, but your heavenly Father already knows all your needs. Seek the Kingdom of God above all else, and live righteously, and he will give you everything you need. So don't worry about tomorrow, for tomorrow will bring its own worries. Today's trouble is enough for today. (Matt. 6:25–34)

Nourish Self

Activity 1: Begin a daily gratitude challenge with an accountability partner.

Write down the simple things in a journal, such as:

- air conditioning on a hot day
- indoor plumbing
- exercise
- books from the library
- hot coffee on a cold day
- funny texts from a friend
- sunshine during a midday walk
- a comfortable bed
- hearing a song you love
- a beautiful sunrise
- phone calls from a loved one
- transportation to work or church

Activity 2: Download a positive affirmations app that sends you a new thought daily on your phone.

Search for apps using phrases like "Christian affirmations" or "daily Christian affirmations" to find ones that may be a good fit.

Activity 3: Make cards with fun and playful activities you want to do or learn.

Enjoy something new and different on an open evening or weekend. For example,

- Learn to play pickleball.
- Take a dance class.
- Play a card game.
- Join a book club.
- Go for a walk with an app that identifies plants and learn about nature.
- Volunteer at the library, pet shelter, or food bank.
- Surprise a person who lives alone with some food and fellowship.
- Learn how to bake bread.
- Sign up for an art class.
- Visit a local museum.
- Be a "tourist" in your own hometown.
- Offer to babysit for friends with young children to give them a date night.

Armor of God

I believe the best way to armor up for the words that we speak or words spoken to us is to spend time reading God's truths.

Consider this verse: "Take the helmet of salvation and the sword of the Spirit, which is the word of God" (Eph. 6:17 NIV).

Since the Word of God is the sword of the Spirit, we can use the truths throughout scripture to cut through the enemy's lies. How does that knowledge change our understanding of spiritual warfare and the role the Word of God plays as a weapon against untruths?

Now, go through each of the scriptures in the "Seek Him" exercise. As you do, ask yourself, *How does this verse combat a lie that the enemy tries to tell me?* Write out your ideas.

Prayer

Dear Lord,

I praise You for Your unending love and faithfulness. Your grace and kindness humble me. Help me to see myself as You see me. Guide my thoughts about myself so that I notice the precious masterpiece You have made in me. Allow me to be filled with Your love, acceptance, and joy so that I overflow with kindness, grace, and mercy to others. Help me to love others well with my words and my heart.
In Your name,

Amen.

CHAPTER 7

Accessorize Your Life

As I parked my car in downtown Paducah to head to an appointment, my mind was in a million places. I felt anxious inside with the weight of decisions, work, logistics, my schedule, and people—so many people—who depend on me. Yet when I tried to do some deep breathing, mindfulness, or prayer—things that typically help me regain peace and bring me into self-awareness—none of them seemed to work. My precious mom and her declining health were simply too heavy a burden. As a physician, our family and everyone else look to me for answers. Despite my education and years of experience in the medical world, I have no answers. Sometimes, there just is not anything medical to do. Sometimes, nature is simply taking its course. Sometimes, acceptance, surrender, and the decision to trust God are the only choices we can make. After all, He alone can hold it all, hear our prayers, and answer according to His will.

As I exited my car and reached the door to the building, I looked up. The sign above the familiar door read "Oh So Beautiful" in a lovely script. *Ahh! A reminder for me.* As I changed into a smock and sat in a black swivel chair, my hairstylist came up behind me. Even though I hadn't said anything, she could tell I needed a hug. She placed her arms around my tired, aching neck and whispered, "Giving you lots of love right now." She had noted the sadness in my eyes and met me with comfort. That is *oh so beautiful* for sure.

There is a phrase we have used in the office, at home with my daughter, or even when I speak to other women that reflects the comfort and confidence we gain from our hair. When having a bad hair day, we quip, "It's not all about the hair," knowing that, well—it really *can* be all about the hair some days. Full disclosure: I am a girl who lived through the 1980s, and there are numerous pictures of me from my younger days where my hair could be counted as another person entirely in the photo.

Whether we are discussing decade-specific hairstyles, makeup trends, or the latest fashions, we gain confidence from many different external variables. These self-imposed and self-evaluated facets of how we look can determine how we feel about ourselves and what we can accomplish throughout the day ahead. Hair is one aspect of that calculation. Beloved, precious ladies who are dealing with hair loss due to chemotherapy, hormonal changes, stress, or a multitude of dermatologic diagnoses desire hope, guidance, treatment, and turban or wig options to regain that part of their beauty.

Along with our hair, our nails and skin are other ways we can complement our beauty, yet they don't represent our true, authentic beauty. Once we find our reflection in Him, we can have fun accessorizing with what brings us joy and let others do the same.

Accessorizing our lives means embellishing ourselves with whatever makes us smile, laugh, feel more confident, and believe that we are beautiful. That embellishment is different for all of us. I have said for years that polka dots and bubbles make me joyful. The bubbles that pop in the air when I squeeze dish soap in the sink are spontaneous, fun moments for me.

Once, when I was taking care of a patient, she complained about the red bumps that kept coming up on her skin.

I explained that they were called angiomas and were a benign, inherited blood vessel type of "mole." She listened to my explanation, then immediately responded by saying how ugly they were and how she hated them. As I smiled and touched her leg, I told her about my love of polka dots and that I had several of these places on my abdomen. Recently, I had decided that God had given me these "polka dots" on my body so that when I looked in the mirror, I saw polka dots and smiled with joy! Perspective makes *such* a difference.

A few weeks later, when the woman returned for a follow-up appointment, I did not remember our dialogue in the exam room, but she did. She said that ever since our appointment, she had started appreciating the fun adornments on her skin and was now actually grateful for them.

A change in perspective can help us embrace everything from unwanted dots on our skin to unexpected challenges, changes, and frustrations in life. This shift in perspective can impact our hearts to live with joy. When our hearts focus on the good in our lives, we live more freely and can sprinkle our joy on others.

These daily interactions with patients reinforce my need to guide them to accurate information about all aspects of their skin. This process is fun for me as I let them guide the discussions. From crepey skin to aging neck skin, makeup dos and don'ts to coconut oil being used for everything, to physical versus chemical sunscreens, accessorizing our skin is simply fun and very individualized.

Cosmetics originated as a play on theatre terms, as actors used them to "make up" themselves as someone else. The focus was on embellishing in order to look better and different. Makeup does not make us, but it can be part of our self-care that enhances our authentic beauty and provides some fun creativity.

Yet, as a dermatologist, I understand the importance of skin health as much more than surface-level cosmetics. This multi-billion-dollar industry of skin care, lotions, and makeup includes plenty of false information. People can spend a lot of money on products recommended on the internet that actually age and impair skin health and vitality.

From skin care to makeup, jewelry to scarves, music to dancing, we can be unapologetically ourselves by accessorizing. In doing so, we embrace creativity and live with joy. This chapter contains information on the correct way to care for skin, protect skin, revitalize skin, and accessorize.

Basics Of Skin Care

Healthy skin is beautiful skin. We can ensure our skin is healthy and vibrant by taking a few minutes every morning and evening to do a few simple steps. As discussed in earlier chapters, our skin reflects our internal health and is impacted by food, exercise, stress management, and sleep. Yet some steps are paramount to care for our skin externally.

My career battles a multi-billion-dollar skincare industry along with DIY products on social media, not to mention free giveaways waiting for you at local malls. I desire to use science to guide people in finding the correct products for their skin to maximize their finances and time budgets most effectively for their skin concerns.

A full skin cell cycle is four to six weeks. This process takes a dividing cell at the base of our top layer of skin through several sub-layers to become a dead, compact skin cell on the top of the skin. For a short period of time, these dead skin cells serve a major function of the skin as the stratum corneum, keeping infection out and hydration in. Then, these dead skin cells slough off as the next layer takes their place.

Even as early as our teen years, this natural exfoliation is hindered. Early on, these dead skin cells get stuck in our hair follicles with increased oil production and begin forming blackheads and whiteheads, potentially leading to acne. Later on, the dead skin cells can stay attached throughout the skin's surface, leading to rough, red, inflamed skin with an irregular texture, roughness, and discoloration or pigmentation.

Proper cleansing, toning, and exfoliation are key to restoring the normal cell cycle. This is accomplished in two basic steps repeated twice daily, with a third step twice weekly: Cleanse, tone, and scrub. Cleansing your skin with a proper cleanser every morning and night removes oil, makeup, pollution, and sweat. This is best accomplished by combining a quality cleanser with warm water and a washcloth or vibrational brush. I do not recommend cleansing wipes, as they leave a residue on the skin. Cleansing wipes can be utilized as a first step for removing the outer layer of makeup and oil but should always be followed by proper cleansing. I recommend splashing warm water on the face first to moisten the skin, applying cleanser and massaging it into the skin with circular movements for sixty seconds, then rinsing with warm water and a washcloth to remove it fully.

Toning the skin must always follow cleansing, as it provides additional exfoliation and helps restore the skin to a proper pH. There are different types of toners available that are typically applied with a pad or spray.

In addition to daily cleansing and toning, using a fine particle scrub two mornings a week allows for additional physical exfoliation of the buildup on the skin. It is helpful for all skin types, even sensitive skin that may be thought not to tolerate a scrub.

Cleansing, toning, and exfoliating are the basic critical steps for healthy skin upkeep and will not take more than two minutes twice a day.

Protection

As a dermatologist who has seen the incidence of skin cancer rise dramatically over the past twenty-five years, sun protection is the next nonnegotiable step. Ultraviolet light (UVL) exposure from sunlight or tanning beds leads to aging of the skin and 98 percent of skin cancers. This includes the ultraviolet light exposure from daily walking in and out of buildings.[1]

We must use sunscreen daily to protect our skin from these damaging rays. I recommend a broad-spectrum sunscreen that protects from UVA and UVB, with an SPF between 30 and 35 for both the face and the body.

It is essential to realize that SPF protection offered in lotions or makeup is insufficient. A true sunscreen should be used before applying makeup. Regarding the specific kind of sunscreen that should be used, both physical and chemical sunscreens are available and are slightly different in their use and benefits. Physical sunscreens contain the active ingredients zinc oxide or titanium dioxide and work by reflecting the UVL rays. They work immediately upon application to the skin and are slightly water-resistant. Chemical sunscreens have true chemicals as their active ingredients. They work by absorbing the

UVL and must be applied before sun exposure, as they require about thirty minutes on the skin before becoming effective. They should be avoided in people with facial rosacea because they heat the skin and increase redness.

All sunscreens are most effective when reapplied every two hours. However, it is important to remember that even the best of sunscreens is not 100 percent effective.[2]

Since Coco Chanel accidentally got too much sun in the French Riviera in the 1920s and arrived home with a tan, tanned skin has been perceived as attractive and desirable in the United States. However, a tan achieved from outdoor ultraviolet light or tanning beds only increases the risk of skin aging and potentially deadly skin cancer. A less risky option is using spray tan or sunless tanning products.

In addition to utilizing sunless tanning products and incorporating a good SPF into your daily routine, you can also protect your skin by wearing ultraviolet protective factor (UPF) clothing. This fabric provides extra protection while active or in the water but remains breathable even in warm temperatures.

Vitamin D

Vitamin D deficiency has been debated and studied extensively in the past decade. The role that sun protection and the use of sunscreen play in this process has been a hot topic—pardon the pun. The bottom line is that we need vitamin D, and we need to protect our skin from the sun. Understanding the facts and dispelling myths about this issue is important because our lives can depend on it.

Vitamin D is essential for bone health. It helps keep our bones strong, decreasing the risk of osteoporosis and bone fractures.

Our immune system is also strengthened when our body has an adequate vitamin D level, helping to prevent infection and several diseases.[3] Therefore, we must find healthy ways to keep our body at an appropriate and necessary level of vitamin D.

Sun protection for our skin is also very important. With that in mind, we must find a way to protect our skin from skin cancer and aging risks as we maintain an appropriate vitamin D level. Here are three common myths about vitamin D:

1. **Sun exposure is the best way to maintain adequate vitamin D.**

   False! The skin is a source of vitamin D. Ultraviolet B rays from the sun react with an aspect of the skin, which is then converted to vitamin D3, the active form of vitamin D.

   The body's ability to convert the inactive to the active form of vitamin D reaches its maximum capacity with just ten to fifteen minutes of sun exposure two to three times a week. After that, the body starts disposing of vitamin D due to overload.[4] The skin as a source of vitamin D is very limited.

2. **Sunscreens prevent the UVB from reaching the skin's surface, effectively stopping natural vitamin D production.**

   False! Since sunscreens do not provide 100 percent protection, some UVB rays will still reach the skin's surface—even when the best sunscreen is used. Studies have failed to show that wearing sunscreen leads to a vitamin D deficiency.[5]

3. **Tanning beds protect against vitamin D deficiency
    and are a safe way to get UVL exposure.**

    False! Tanning beds utilize UVA light, which causes
    premature skin aging, brown discoloration, and deeper
    penetration into the skin that causes cell damage and
    increases the risk of skin cancer. People who use indoor
    tanning beds are 74 percent more likely to develop
    melanoma than those who do not use tanning beds.
    They are also 2.5 times more likely to get squamous cell
    cancer and 1.5 times more likely to get basal cell cancer.[6]

    In addition, the light rays used by tanning beds do
    not include UVB, which is the ultraviolet ray that can
    convert inactive vitamin D to active vitamin D, result-
    ing in no additional natural production of vitamin D.[7]

    UVA also weakens the immune system, adding
    to the risk of disease created by having a vitamin D
    deficiency.[8]

Instead of falling into the trap of believing false information, seek sources of vitamin D that will improve your health
and provide an adequate amount of this important vitamin. To
optimize your health with adequate vitamin D levels and protect
your skin from skin cancer and aging, get vitamin D from your
foods (such as fatty fish or fortified foods such as orange juice),
supplements, and incidental sun exposure. The Institute of Medicine recommends 600 IU of vitamin D daily for most people.[9]

Hydration

Our skin possesses the natural moisturizing factor (NMF) to
maintain adequate skin hydration. This allows our skin to

maintain its proper texture and the skin barrier. However, due to environmental factors as well as the normal aging process, at some point, we need to make sure we begin adding effective moisturizers to the skin. Many over-the-counter lotions and moisturizers for the face and body are large-molecule products that are not absorbed into the skin to hydrate effectively. They sit on top of the skin, making it feel better for a short period but eventually leading to further dryness, inflammation, and inhibition of our NMF.

To aid the body's ability to absorb moisture, I recommend using a dry brushing technique before showering or bathing. This aids in exfoliating dead skin cells that prevent effective moisturizers from properly absorbing. Dry brushing involves taking a boar bristle brush and brushing skin from the feet and hands toward the heart. After showering or bathing, simply towel dry and apply an effective body lotion that does not contain fragrance and is approved by a dermatologist.

For the face, I recommend using a quality medical-grade product with hyaluronic acid as one of the main ingredients.

After starting this routine, stay consistent. Avoid the distractions of social media and advertising that draw you away from your routine. Most trendy recommendations are temporary and not proven to work over time. For instance, while coconut oil is natural, it is not an effective way to hydrate your skin.

The microbiome conversation—regarding the natural bacteria in our gut and skin—has been incredibly powerful over the last few years, with excellent research guiding recommendations. Just as our gut microbiome has been found to impact our health greatly and requires support by eating fruits and vegetables and minimizing inflammatory foods, the skin microbiome must be supported as well to maintain its proper function and look. This is accomplished externally with proper exfoliation, hydration, and barrier repair maintenance, as discussed. Some products specifically address restoring the skin microbiome, such as Avenue Thermal Spring Water, which can be used as a spritz daily.

Revitalization

Revitalization is defined as imbuing something with new life and vitality.[10] That is a beautiful word picture of our life in Christ and how His tender mercies are new every morning. Let's pause for a minute in the midst of finding a few daily steps that we can take to maintain healthy skin and remember the God who defines and supplies our new life and vitality. Ah, yes!

Just as guilt, fear, rejection, shame, and other negative emotions can get stuck in our hearts and minds, day-to-day living and aging get in and on our skin. Thankfully, specific options are available to address the problems we see. This part of skin care becomes more tailored to individual needs.

Here are a few of the most common issues:

- For large pores, blackheads, whiteheads, and fine lines on the face, we need to add a product that stimulates cell turnover. This is a prescription-strength Retin-A cream or OTC retinol. I highly recommend choosing a product recommended by a trusted source— such as a dermatologist or an aesthetician—as many on the market are not of adequate quality.

- For additional dryness, aging, and inflammation on the facial skin, using a hyaluronic acid, collagen, or peptide cream is helpful.

- For irregular pigment and brown skin spots, combinations of bleaching and blending creams need to be rotated on and off the skin.

Makeup

Although makeup does not make us, it can be embraced to accentuate our natural beauty. When we choose which makeup to use, it's best to keep it simple.

Here's a quick overview of a makeup routine to help you feel good inside and out. As you complete each item, spend time meditating on God's Word.

> **Foundation:** Choose a light, mineral-based liquid foundation for easy application, then set it with a loose powder.
> Ponder the following verses:
>
> ✝ Instruct them to do good, to be rich in good works, to be generous and ready to share, storing up for themselves the treasure of a good foundation for the future, so that they may take hold of that which is truly life. (1 Tim. 6:18–19 NASB 1995)
>
> ✝ Just as He chose us in Him before the foundation of the world, that we would be holy and blameless before him. (Eph. 1:4)
>
> **Contour:** Contouring the skin occurs when you use bronzer, blush, and highlighter or illumination sticks to define the cheeks and angles of the face. Bronzer

can be applied on both sides of our cheeks below the cheekbone, and then a little blush can be added to the center of the cheek. Applying an illumination stick or highlighter works well for the lower rim of the eye near the crow's feet area and sides of the nose.

Think about how to let your light shine as you illuminate the paths of those around you with joy throughout the day ahead.

Eye shadow and eyeliner: Trends and seasons change quickly for eye shadow and application techniques. I encourage my patients to watch YouTube videos to accomplish the most up-to-date looks.

As you apply your eye makeup, say Hebrews 12:2, "fixing our eyes on Jesus, the author and perfected of our faith, who for the joy set before him endured the cross, scorning its shame, and sat down at the right hand of the throne of God."

Eyebrows: Our eyebrows shape our face, and using an eyebrow pencil can add further definition. Most newer eyebrow pencils offer excellent feathering options for those with thinning eyebrows.

Consider how your life is defined according to 1 Peter 2:9: "But you are a chosen race, a royal priesthood, a holy nation, a people for his own possession, that you may proclaim the excellencies of him who called you out of darkness into his marvelous light."

Lips: Like eye shadow and eyeliner techniques, lip colors are also driven by current trends. Which color is in style, whether a matte or glossy look is desirable, and whether or not to use lipliner is often up for debate. However, I find this to be a matter of personal preference. Use what you like and enjoy. If you choose not to use color on your lips, I recommend applying a lip balm with an SPF of at least 15 in the morning to decrease the risk of skin cancer developing later in life. Also, use a quality lip balm at night to keep lips hydrated.

As you apply a product to your lips, be reminded to season your words with grace. Extend love, joy, and kindness all day long.

Adding our personal style to life is what keeps it interesting. Fashion and makeup trends can guide our choices, but, ultimately, we should pick the things that make us feel like the best version of ourselves.

Accessorize

After taking care of our skin, what does it look like to accessorize? Once we have established in our hearts that we *are* beautiful, let's embrace the desires of our hearts. Embody your quirky, authentic, fun self through clothing, scarves, jewelry, purses, hairstyles, shoes, and more. We can trust the promise of Psalms 37:4–5: "Delight yourself in the LORD; . . . Trust also in Him, and He will do it." If you love art, seek out ways to create and view art. If you love music, join me as I dance in my car, listening to Christian music. If you love to grow plants or flowers, start a garden or volunteer in a community garden. If you make a food choice that feels like a splurge, have no guilt—it is a choice, not a cheat. Simply accept it and move on.

As you will read in the next chapter, red is a significant color to my mother and me. I have very few vivid memories of when

I was three, but one is etched permanently in my mind. I had a red pair of shoes that I loved to wear. I also had a favorite red skirt. I would ask to wear both often, even if they were dirty or not appropriate to wear for the activity of the day. However, one Sunday morning, as my mother was getting my younger brother ready for church, I asked her if I could wear my red skirt and shoes. She said yes. I put them on and took my place in a small rocking chair in the living room next to my older sister, where we were told to wait until it was time to leave. As I rocked myself in the chair, I remember thinking, *I am so cute!*

We all have experienced joy when everything falls into place, and we can enjoy the moment. Our heart feels full and ready to overflow because of our confidence in ourselves. Sometimes, this is simply a choice that we make despite our circumstances. We know life will never be devoid of pain, challenges, struggles, grief, or heartache. That is why I love to reflect on the verse that my company is named after: "Above all else, guard your heart, for it is the wellspring of life" (Prov. 4:23 NIV). We can guard, guide, and protect our hearts by filling ourselves up with God's Word and His truths about how beautifully we were created.

One real beauty of adorning your life is to live it out for others. Some of my most joyful moments have occurred when volunteering for the sake of others. Serving others helps take the focus off our trials, the challenges ahead, and the difficulties we face in this season of life by demonstrating opportunities for us to do something for someone else. Consider pausing amid your morning routine and ask God to show you a few simple things you can do today for someone He places in your path. Following His lead will bring richness to your soul and strength to your stride.

SNAP

Seek Him

Seek His truths to recognize the unique aspects of who you are and what you desire or what brings you joy. Then, live out your beautiful self unapologetically.

MEDITATE ON THESE WORDS

✟ For we are God's handiwork, created in Christ Jesus to do good works, which God prepared in advance for us to do. (Eph. 2:10)

✟ Finally, brothers and sisters, Whatever is true, whatever is noble, whatever is right, whatever is pure, whatever is lovely, whatever is admirable, if anything is excellent or praiseworthy, think on such things. (Phil. 4:8)

✟ I also want the women to dress modestly, with decency and propriety, adorning themselves, not with elaborate hairstyles or gold or pearls or expensive clothes, but with good deeds, appropriate for women who profess to worship God. (1 Tim. 2:9–10)

✝ Charm is deceptive, and beauty is fleeting; but a woman who fears the Lord is to be praised. (Prov. 31:30)

✝ Delight yourself in the LORD; and He will give you the desires of your heart. (Ps. 37:4 NASB 1995)

✝ So Jesus said to the Jews who had believed Him, "If you abide in My word, then you are truly My disciples; and you will know the truth, and the truth will set you free." (John 8:31–32 ESV)

Nourish Self

Nourish yourself with the fun things in life. Do those things that lead to a belly laugh, a childlike twinkle in your eye, or joy in your soul. Remember when you were a child and lived out of that place of wonder? Notice the beauty around you and share it with others. Consider grabbing an accountability partner for a month or two at a time and sending each other a daily message noting three beautiful things.

Implement healthy skincare practices:

- Take two minutes every morning and evening to cleanse and tone your skin, adding a scrub two mornings a week.

- Use daily sunscreen on all the skin exposed to the sun that day.

- Tailor additional skincare products according to your specific needs, such as lightening dark spots, improving overall texture or redness, minimizing fine lines and wrinkles, and hydrating dry and inflamed skin. For specific recommendations on quality products, I encourage you to go to my website and take the skincare assessment.

- Exfoliate skin with a dry brush before showering and apply moisturizer after toweling dry.

Armor of God

When we read about putting our armor on in Ephesians 6, we are given the example of pieces of clothing. These symbolic reminders encourage us to look at God's provisions for the day, accompanying us each day as a part of our outfit. As you choose your makeup, clothing, jewelry, and other accessories for the day, ponder how they make you unique. Think of how they make you feel. Enjoy sharing a little of yourself in how you look.

Accessorize yourself:

- Add lip color for the day.

- Polish your nails.

- Find a new way to use a scarf as an accessory.

- Find a place to volunteer in your community this month.

- Plant a small garden of flowers or vegetables.

- Go to your local hobby store and consider learning to paint.

- Whatever causes your insides to come alive, do it.

Prayer

Dear Lord,

THANK YOU FOR THE SPECIAL WAY YOU INTRICATELY MADE me. Help me embrace my uniqueness and unapologetically live how You intended me to. Guide my choices for accessorizing my life. May I seek to use opportunities that arise and the many blessings in my life to serve those You put in my path today. Let me embrace my worth fully in You, so the freedom and abundance I gain is for Your glory.
In Jesus's name,

Amen.

CHAPTER 8

All Eyes on Us

I TOOK A DEEP BREATH TO CALM MY FEARS WHILE WALKING up the dirt road alongside security guards with my husband and three children. It was our first day in Honduras. As I glanced around and noticed children of all ages kicking a soccer ball on the grassy slope of the mountain—shoeless, with dirty faces and contagious laughter—my shoulders began to drop. I caught my breath as my spirit settled. I became lost in the moment as I noticed people of all ages gratefully welcoming us to this small village. I had a deep desire to capture the images of those around me.

As my adult children will attest, I love to take pictures. In their younger years, their annoyance didn't stop me from doing so. But on this mountain in Honduras, my photography skills were appreciated in a refreshing new way. I pulled out my camera to capture these amazingly resilient people and received quite a different reaction from the children and adults than my own children. Instead of annoyance, the residents immediately surrounded me and smiled, wanting their picture taken.

Now perched at the top of the mountain, I paused to stare off into the beautiful green countryside. We were visiting a remote Honduran village, and despite the lovely surroundings, I couldn't help but question God. I could not make sense of the vast difference between my home in Kentucky—with its stocked refrigerator, air-conditioning, comfortable bed, and all the comforts of modern living in the US—and compare it to this tiny mountainside village in Honduras, where most of the residents did not have a legitimate roof over their heads and slept on dirt floors.

The trip had sprung from a deep desire to take our children on mission work to instill a servant's heart and help them recognize that they led an extremely comfortable life. My husband and I, as physicians, spent our days that week seeing patients. Our sons helped the construction crew build housing for some of the local people, while our daughter worked in the makeshift pharmacy to dispense medications we had been collecting for more than a year. Each day began with an early morning devotional at the hotel, followed by a harrowing trip up the mountain on an ancient bus. The dirt road would eventually get so rough that we would walk the final mile to the village where the day's work began.

As I talked to God on that mountaintop, a rush of guilt ran through me. Yes, I was there that week to help with medical care for people who typically had no access to simple pain relievers for their toothaches, joint aches, or headaches. But was I really making a difference? I wanted to know deep in my spirit that we were truly providing lasting care, comfort, and impact. Yet I felt so inadequate.

There is one child I will never forget. She was about ten years old with dark brown hair, tired eyes, a green shirt, and a precious smile. She came into the clinic to see us and let us know through the interpreter that she had a sore throat. When I asked her to open her mouth so that I could look at her throat, I saw five large, abscessed teeth with very swollen gums. When the interpreter asked if her teeth and gums hurt, she looked at me and nodded yes. Even a toothache blunted by ibuprofen or acetaminophen feels awful. But the pain this sweet girl lived with took my breath away. I had to turn away for a moment, tears in my eyes, as I considered the immense pain she faced daily.

Despite all the people we were able to assist that week, I still found myself asking God: *Did we make any difference?*

Even now, that question remains at the forefront of my heart and mind. I am flooded with questions when I crawl into bed and lay my head on my pillow each night. *Was I a good mom today, and now, as a grandmother, a good "Mimi"? Did I care for all my patients with discernment and compassion? Did I support the incredible women who work for me? Did I use kind words throughout my day? Did I see—truly see—people and love them well throughout my day? Did I care for the neighbor in my path? Was I fully present as a wife, sister, and friend? Did I extend grace to myself?* I want to know that I served God well that day. I want to know that Jesus says, "Evelyn, you did great today." I want to know I'm pleasing to Him.

Though I've always wanted to use my life to serve God, the trip was a reminder of that priority.

Most of our discussion throughout this book has been about recognizing and valuing our beauty. But as Christians, we can use what we've learned to mentor those around us.

Ambassadors for Jesus

When my mother was the mayor of Paducah, Kentucky, she wore red. As a retired schoolteacher, her intention wasn't to draw attention to herself but to promote tourism in the area. She began an ambassador program to get river steamboats to make Paducah one of their ports of call. The volunteer program educated "Paducahans" about their community, gave them a red jacket, and had them provide tours, directions, and information to tourists. Thirty-two years later, the program has logged more than eighty thousand volunteer hours. The purpose of choosing a red jacket—and for my mother to wear red clothes as the mayor—was to encourage the ambassadors to stand out.

When we follow Jesus, we choose to have eyes on us. As ambassadors for Christ, we may not wear red, but we are clothed in Him. Even as we learn to focus on our many blessings, we will become free to wow the world with our servant hearts. Serving is the best way to exemplify the love of Jesus to others. In each season of life, let's live for Him without comparison, regret, cynicism, or what-ifs holding us back. Instead, let's put our influence and opportunities to good use.

I was fortunate to have been modeled a servant's heart by both parents. They were both mission-driven, service-minded people, so that is what I assumed I should do from an early age. They were my first mentors.

About eighteen years before my mother died, she became ill with a life-threatening heart issue. Doctors gave her less than a 10 percent chance of living through the required surgery. As her family, we remained alongside her—by her hospital bed, through her rehabilitation work, and as she transitioned home—observing her sheer determination to make it. She did! A few days after returning home in January 2004, she received the Chamber of Commerce Annual Community Service Award.

I accepted the award on her behalf, telling the crowd: "I know she would want me to say that it is because of the work of so many of you here that she has accomplished much of what she has in community service. She is recuperating at home and is anxious to return to service in this community with all of you."

My mother was keenly aware that our individual service is vital in accomplishing our collective goals. Eleanor Roosevelt, a courageous advocate of service to others, once said, "We should rejoice in the accomplishments of those before us, be proud of the heritage that we inherit, but be always vigilant that the future is ours alone to make."[1]

To me, my mother was the Eleanor Roosevelt of Paducah. She tirelessly and unselfishly worked in her community to make it a better place to live. And in doing so, she encouraged others to follow her example.

As Philippians 2:3–4 (NASB 1995) reminds us, "Do nothing from selfishness or empty conceit, but with humility of mind let each of you regard one another as more important than himself; do not merely look out for your own personal interests, but also for the interests of others."

When we choose to serve, other people notice. But although we often think of service as something active that we do physically—feeding those who are hungry, caring for those who are sick or in need, or volunteering in our community—our influence extends far beyond our list of activities.

One of the most underappreciated forms of service is mentorship. Mentoring others doesn't sound flashy, and it isn't. Although someone might be lauded for raising vast sums of money for a worthy cause, a mentor can be easily overlooked. Yet their quiet one-on-one interactions may be just as life-changing.

Mentoring Others

Two women in their mid-twenties called me one Sunday afternoon on their way home from church in another city. They were worked up and needed to vent about a message they wanted to ensure I included in my talks and writings.

Both had been raised in church from a young age and attended a ladies' Sunday school class that morning.

The woman who was teaching started by introducing herself. She was one of the elder's wives and had been in church her entire life. Much older than these two younger women, she said she wasn't sure she was qualified to teach but would try.

How demoralizing! The young women told me, "If she isn't qualified, we will never be." They understood her heart and desire, but it brought a sense of perfectionism that they knew they would never attain.

Our attempt at humility and meekness can sometimes be such a discouragement to others. As we are told in 2 Timothy 1:7, "God does not give us a spirit of timidity, but of power and love and discipline."

God placed us on the earth in this era for His work and a purpose (our "such a time as this"), and He will equip us to accomplish it.

It's true that this world is not the same one I grew up in—some things are better, some worse. But younger generations need to hear messages of empowerment, trust, confidence, and hope from us. They don't need doom, gloom, or relentless nostalgia for the old days. They don't need us to lump them in with other people their age, make assumptions about who they are, or tell them, "I am glad I am not your age or raising my kids now."

Instead, let's use our influence to encourage them.

A woman in her late fifties told me how much her views on marriage and motherhood had shifted over time, saying, "I believe in my younger years, I had a distorted view of what marriage and motherhood were supposed to look like. Though sacrifice is necessary, it isn't a badge of honor. By learning to care for myself during those years, I could have better modeled what that would look like for my children."

The truth is that life experience has value, and younger women need this message of encouragement and perspective that only we can provide. One thing I have heard from older women is the idea that it's someone else's turn. It's a younger woman's turn to carry the torch. Yet our faith is often compared to a race—not a sprint, but a long, slow path toward obedience.

Galatians 5:7 (ESV) reminds us of the importance of pursuing God, regardless of age or situation. In it, Paul asks an all-important question: "You were running well. Who hindered you from obeying the truth?" There is no expiration date to following God's will.

Mentoring Faith

Statistics show the church loses four to six out of every ten people we baptize.[2] As Christians, we must plant seeds, but we also need to encourage those who are Christians to grow beyond the milk of the word because we need God's wisdom to navigate this world.

We tend to think of mentoring as an older-to-younger transfer of wisdom, but mentoring can go both ways, especially when it comes to our faith. We can glean a lot from those older than us and those younger than us. Christians in their forties need just as much encouragement as those in their twenties or those in their sixties. Age does not make us immune from the challenges of life.

The wonderful thing about faith is that it is not static. As we continue to learn, our faith grows and shifts. Faith leads us on a grand adventure that never ends.

That does not mean it is an adventure devoid of struggle or hardship. But by being authentic in our faith journey—allowing others to see us wrestle with God about how and why bad things happen to the faithful—we can demonstrate how to be faithful despite and amid the questions, pain, struggle, and fight.

Reading and understanding scripture is one of the most powerful ways we mature in our faith. We begin as 1 Peter 2:2 (NIV) describes: "Like newborn babies, crave pure spiritual milk, so that by it you may grow up in your salvation," but we move toward spiritual maturity and discernment over time.

Our belief systems guide our choices in life, and if our ultimate goal is to continually grow in our faith and understanding of God's Word, then our choices will naturally evolve. When they do, we can use our newfound knowledge to encourage and mentor others.

In Cleo Wade's book, *Remember Love: Words for Tender Times*, there is a poem titled "everything that's happened":

> there are some very large letting goes to do:
> people, places, honeyed and bitter phases of life
> there are some even larger letting goes to do:
> angers, tears, parts of yourself that leave with no return
>
> have a past
>
> everything that's happened cannot be held today.[3]

This idea resonates with me in a powerful and personal way. I have wanted to please God since I was a young girl, yet I have made many mistakes and missteps. I wish I had handled all interactions with others along my journey with grace and discernment, allaying regret. But that is simply not true. I have made choices that were not true to who I am in Christ, and for that, I am remorseful. There have been times when I did not let the light of my faith shine and instead let Satan win the battle of my words and actions. So I desire grace to be extended to me. I desire those who have witnessed me in those situations not to presume that is who I am presently. Understanding this for myself helps me also appreciate that the same is true for others. Acknowledging wherever we are on this life journey, we can close the windows and mirrors of comparison and see what is true and authentic right now.

Let's have the strength to trust God with others' faith journey, speak the truth, and love them. Let's show others that we have confidence in them.

We can guide and empower without shame or comparisons but with knowledge, understanding, and love. Many times, that comes down to how we say things.

Instead of saying, "You should" (i.e., "You should always be at church"), let's turn the conversation into a dialogue. Consider how these phrases sound:

- "Tell me what your challenges are right now."

- "Tell me what obstacles Satan is putting in your path to slow your growth in faith and trust."

- "Consider this . . ."

- "How can I pray for you to encourage you and lighten your load?"

"Should" messages convey that the other person has messed up, and we believe it's our job to tell them how to fix it. Our language can promote courage and a desire to live our best life or provoke shame and hopelessness.

Instead, ask others, "What is God doing in your life right now?" And when you see someone living out their faith, uplift them with this truth: "God sure does look good on you." That, friends, is true beauty.

What Service Looks Like

I just recently returned from the International Plant-Based Nutrition Healthcare Conference in California, listening to the latest research and studies about how the types of foods we eat and how we live our life impacts every aspect of our health. The speakers included cardiologists, gastroenterologists, internists, lifestyle medicine physicians, nutritionists, and those with a PhD in public health. The information was relevant, timely, and powerful, yet it was simplistic in many ways. The same lifestyle choices—including healthy eating, stress management, daily movement or exercise, and proper sleep—improve all aspects of health. Yet the foundation of optimal health and quality of life is having a sense of purpose and meaning. Even a Blue Zones documentary on Netflix discussed how having a purpose and reason to get up every day brings deep, abundant joy and leads to healthier choices in other areas of our lives. A sense of purpose is vital to our health.[4]

When we live for a purpose outside of ourselves—whether serving others or showing care and respect toward nature—we gain meaning and richness in our lives. It can feel like we need to do something big or significant to make an impact. However, using Jesus as our mentor, we simply choose to be aware of those around us and serve in the moments we are given, just as Jesus demonstrated healing and encouragement as He walked throughout His day. We can also intentionally mentor others, just as Jesus did when teaching His twelve apostles.

Daily Service

When I stood up to say a few words at our daughter's rehearsal dinner, I felt an overwhelming sense of gratitude as I looked out at the faces of close family and friends alongside new faces we had welcomed into our family. I told them that our time is one of the greatest gifts we can give. We all have many things that demand a spot on our calendar, yet at some point, we choose what we will show up for and turn our attention toward. By celebrating our daughter that evening, I knew people had made sacrifices, said no to other things, and spent their money to be with us that weekend. It touched my heart and brought me to tears.

Our daily act of service can be as simple as giving our time to a need that we have noticed. We choose to be content with our current circumstances and find a way to give and serve from there.

Loneliness has become an epidemic that affects all of us. Three in five Americans report feeling lonely, and nearly a quarter of those sixty-five and older are considered socially isolated. Loneliness can also negatively impact health by increasing the rate of dementia and heart disease, decreasing our functionality as we age, and leading to earlier death.[5]

Thankfully, serving others is one of the best ways to combat loneliness. About two-thirds of respondents in a British study agreed that volunteering had helped them feel less isolated, especially for those ages eighteen to thirty-four.[6] This sense of well-being as a result of serving others rings true for older adults, as well: AARP Foundation Experience Corps found that more than 85 percent of volunteers felt their lives had improved because of their involvement with the program, and 98 percent said it helped them stay physically and mentally active.[7] Experts say that volunteering not only helps people feel less lonely but can also improve physical well-being.[8] A five-year study found that helping people who don't live with you can act as a buffer against the adverse effects of stress. Although participants encountered stressful life events, those who spent time doing tasks for others were less likely to die than those who had not.[9] Caring for others is truly a way to care for ourselves, as well.

There is no formula or precise picture of daily service or what it looks like. However, when we meet a need right in front of us, then we are serving. It reminds me of a commercial on television that documented random acts of kindness and demonstrated how they are contagious to those who observe them. Doing something for someone else without expecting anything in return enriches our lives with emotions far more powerful than any monetary compensation.

So let's begin to look around and find opportunities in our day-to-day lives that bless others. In the end, we will be the ones truly blessed. A door held open, a tender smile, an errand run, a short visit over coffee, groceries delivered, a listening ear—the list goes on and on. Maybe you offer to trade off carpool or child pick-up, babysit for a couple to have a night out, or stop to see someone who doesn't get many visitors.

Serving people is the most important kind of service we can carry out. But we also have an obligation and opportunity to care for and have a servant's heart for our planet. This kind of daily service can impact those around us, even if it's simply beautifying our surroundings. From simple things like not littering to considering ways to recycle, we can leave every encounter (with people, our community, and our planet) better than we find them. For example, I noticed no litter or trash on a recent Slovenia trip. When we asked our local guide about the clean surroundings, he said that children are taught from kindergarten that if you have trash, put it in the trash bin. Simple! Yet we may need to be taught and mentored in caring for our environment and people. Demonstrating those ideas can be one more act of service we implement regularly.

Each time you choose to pause and serve somehow, take a moment to center yourself in contentment, grateful for the opportunity. Doing so helps us be more truly present, which is deeply felt by those we encounter.

Intentional Mentoring

Several years before my parents passed away, they traveled to Israel. There were many highlights, but what I remember the most when they returned was their description of a wood carving they purchased. It arrived a few weeks later after being shipped to the US. It was a four-by-two-foot carving from acacia wood of Jesus washing an apostle's feet. Though they were donating it to their church to be placed in the foyer, they had a smaller replica made for their home. I was mesmerized by this piece as it reflected Jesus's immense compassion and heart for serving, evidenced by this detailed carving of an intentional moment in Jesus's ministry.

I believe Jesus's decision to wash his apostles' feet was a powerful example of His humility and desire to mentor His disciples in serving and loving others. He wanted them—and now us—to see that our time on this earth can be spent intentionally choosing to guide, empower, and mentor those who are younger in their faith to love and serve as Jesus did. This is the message of Titus 2:3–5:

> Likewise, teach the older women to be reverent in
> the way they live, not to be slanderers or addicted to
> much wine, but to teach what is good. Then they can
> urge the younger women to love their husbands and
> children, to be self-controlled and pure, to be busy at
> home, to be kind, and to be subject to their husbands,
> so that no one will malign the word of God.

I love how Susan Hunt frames the important, powerful work of mentoring others: "Women need women who will share their lives to train them how to apply the Word to all of life—how to love others, care for their families, cultivate community, work productively, and extend compassion according to God's Word."[10]

Unfortunately, many of us have fallen for the lie that we are not needed as mentors. But the truth is that we are always mentoring and modeling! Whether we mean to or not, the words we speak, actions we take, and attitudes we use to approach life ripple out to those around us, including our children, grandchildren, other women, teens, and girls that we influence.

That's why it's so important that when it comes to physical, mental, emotional, and spiritual health, we must start by putting effort into our health and well-being. Let's ask ourselves: *What am I modeling to my daughter, niece, or friend about my worth or theirs if I do not choose self-care?* When we show younger girls that we love ourselves enough to care for ourselves, we demonstrate that as God's children—wholly and deeply loved— we are worthy of seeking wholeness. We need not apologize for being lifelong learners in caring for ourselves.

When it comes to our health, the concept of fake-it-till-you-make-it has some credibility. As lifelong learners, we can choose a method and format that works for us. Listen to podcasts, audio-books, or scripture when doing chores or driving. Making wise choices to care for ourselves requires discipline, but it is worth it. Let's claim our brain health and learn. Doing so empowers us and impacts those around us, whether we realize it or not.

Even when we begin to care for ourselves, we often encounter barriers to intentional mentoring. Many of us feel uncomfortable stepping into a mentor role. Some of the most common barriers I hear include:

- The season of life we're in, whether we are moms of young children or older people with mobility issues or health limitations.

- An overly cluttered, busy schedule that doesn't have time for anything else.

- A failure to act when we feel the nudge. We want to do something for others, but it's easier to think "someone else will do that."

- The worry that we don't know enough.

Can I tell you that all of these barriers have solutions? For instance, if your season of life makes meeting with another person difficult, can you mentor someone by consistently praying for and with them? Can you send them a text with a written-out prayer to encourage them? Prayer costs us nothing and can uplift others no matter our circumstances.

If we have an overly busy life, we can review our schedule and ask ourselves: *Have I said yes to something I now regret? Do we need to continue this activity? Have my priorities shifted since I agreed to this activity? What is God calling me to do in this season of life?* I love how Gary Henry challenges us to reconsider how we spend our time: "God's work requires us to be engaged in life's activities, but growing deep roots in God's character requires solitude and silence."[11]

If we have difficulty obeying the Holy Spirit's nudge, let's commit ourselves to starting small. Perhaps we can double our meal to share half of it with someone else, ask someone out for coffee to see what God is doing in their lives, send a note in the mail, stop by to check on or pray with someone who is housebound, or take the trash can back to the house so a family member doesn't need to.

Yet even if we can overcome all these barriers, many of us have the silent fear that we don't know enough when it comes to spiritual mentoring. Someone else knows the Bible better than we do, can find the scripture more quickly, or has been a Christian longer. Thankfully, God is not put off by what we consider weaknesses, including any knowledge we don't yet have. As Charles Stanley reminds us, "He gives you His energy, wisdom, and strength to fulfill His purposes and make you fruitful for His kingdom."[12]

When we rely on the Holy Spirit, He will give us the words to encourage others. As you've probably heard, God doesn't call the equipped; He equips the called.

Fruit is used as an analogy for serving others throughout scripture. In this case, our ability to bear fruit reflects our faithfulness to the work He has called us to accomplish. When Ephesians 4:1 references the call God has placed on our lives—"As a prisoner for the Lord, then, I urge you to live a life worthy of the calling you have received"—it is clear that we are called to action.

How can we pursue God's call and bear fruit in our lives? After all, Luke 10 tells us that while the work is plentiful, the workers are few. Gary Henry asks us to consider an essential question in his book, *Diligently Seeking God.* "What does God desire from us? Surely he desires our hands, as well as our hearts."[13]

The idea is clear: We are not merely witnesses of God's Kingdom but active participants in the ongoing work. As John 15:8 (ESV) reminds us, "By this my Father is glorified, that you bear much fruit and so prove to be my disciples." Here, "fruit" is something that we produce—evidence not only of our desire to share the Good News of Jesus (producing the fruit of our labor) but also that we are growing in our relationship with Him (evidenced by the fruits of the Spirit in our lives).

Thankfully, you and I can determine many things, including our calendar and commitments. Let's take the time to reevaluate what we spend our time doing. When we reset our priorities to focus on growing spiritually and serving others, we may need to say no to a few things. But when we consciously embrace our role as a worker for the Lord, you—and all those you serve or mentor—will be blessed!

SNAP

Seek Him

As you seek Him, ask God to show you how to use your life to truly see and serve those in your path every day.

MEDITATE ON THESE WORDS

✝ Therefore, knowing the fear of the Lord, we persuade men, but we are made manifest to God; and I hope that we are made manifest also in your consciences. . . . Therefore, we are ambassadors for Christ, as though God were making an appeal through us; we beg you on behalf of Christ, be reconciled to God. (2 Cor. 5:11, 20 NASB 1995)

✝ For which I am an ambassador in chains; that in proclaiming it I may speak boldly, as I ought to speak. (Eph. 6:20)

✝ From Zion, perfect in beauty, God shines forth. (Ps. 50:2 KJV)

✝ But the fruit of the Spirit is love, joy, peace, patience, kindness, goodness, faithfulness . . . (Gal. 5:22 ESV)

✝ Iron sharpens iron, and one man sharpens another. (Prov. 27:17)

✝ One generation shall commend your works to another, and shall declare your mighty acts. (Ps. 145:4)

✝ Be imitators of me, as I am of Christ. (1 Cor. 11:1)

✝ The unfolding of your words gives light; it imparts understanding to the simple. (Ps. 119:130 NIV)

✝ Let the word of Christ dwell in you richly, teaching and admonishing one another in all wisdom, singing psalms and hymns and spiritual songs, with thankfulness in your hearts to God. (Col. 3:16 ESV)

Nourish Self

Now that we've discussed the importance of mentoring, spend time today asking yourself: *Whom can I mentor spiritually, and whom can I serve physically?*

Remember that our mentoring is not tied to spiritual growth or outcomes. God is in charge of the growth. We are simply available to share His wisdom from our perspective and life.

This can take the form of more structured service and mentoring as we make ourselves available to meet with, pray for, and study alongside women who are not necessarily chronologically younger but younger in their faith.

Practically speaking, this can be anything from asking others how we can pray for them to regularly meeting in person or by phone, checking in, and seeing how they navigate challenges. Or it can involve picking a particular subject or book of the Bible to study together and setting a time to meet to review and discuss. It may also take the form of teaching a Bible class at church. Another possibility is to use this book as a group study and meeting to discuss the SNAP challenges.

Here are several important tips:

- Make yourself available to be a mentor, yet set limits based on what your calendar can handle. Remember, overextending yourself will not accomplish the good God intends. So say yes to the opportunities you know you can reasonably complete and fulfill them well.

- Set the planned time for mentorship: how frequently and for what duration.

- Set limitations on your availability or access when giving out your contact information.

Armor of God

The armor of God is not physical armor but spiritual armor. As we clothe ourselves in Christ, we invite others to watch us navigate challenges, rudeness, unfair treatment, and injustice. Our nonverbal communication can be loud to those around us. As Ephesians 6:12 reminds us, we mentor others by acknowledging and accepting that the people in front of us are not the true source of our struggles. Instead, there is a spiritual war going on. When we face darkness, we must understand that while people may hurt us, we are not fighting them. Instead, we are fighting evil.

As we face ourselves in the mirror each day, we must align the breastplate of righteousness with the helmet of salvation. Focusing on these heavenly attributes reminds us that our time here is temporary.

Our daily armor (the truths of God's Word) helps us stay connected to Jesus as our root and source of stability and enables us to exemplify and model the fruits of the spirit.

Prayer

DEAR HEAVENLY FATHER,

*H*ELP ME TO PAUSE IN THE MIDST OF MY DAYS, TO SPEND time with You and Your truths so that I produce the fruits of Your spirit. Allow things and people to see how I am on Your anvil and potter's wheel, ready to be molded and pruned for Your work and glory.

Help me to stay so connected to You that I can follow Paul's example, causing others to imitate and follow the example of a life lived for You (1 Cor. 4:16).

I am awed by the many people You have placed in my life to demonstrate Your grace and mercy. I am indebted to them and to You to live this precious life honoring and embracing their example. Give me people to teach about Your truths and hope. When I feel inadequate, give me words to speak seasoned with grace.

Give me eyes to see and ears to hear the needs of those around me so that my heart will lead me to act in kindness and service to others.

In Jesus's name,

Amen.

CHAPTER 9

Come to the Well

*W*HAT DO WE DO WHEN WE ARE TIRED, WEARY, AND cannot seem to choose the next right thing? In those moments—when we realize we have let the world influence our heart, mind, soul, or body—we must choose to return to Jesus.

The story of the woman at the well (John 4) sums up life's journey in a beautiful, visual way. This precious woman was physically thirsty, tired, isolated, lived for other people's attention, and did not know Jesus. She felt unworthy even to be seen by Him. Yet she was curious about how He could give her water, wanted to know what was so different about His water, and longed to understand why she needed that type of water. She leaned in. She listened. She took time to hear Him and discovered hope in the process.

The woman at the well left the encounter changed, on a mission to tell everyone about who He was. Those few moments with Jesus transformed her pain into hope, and nothing could stop her from living out His commission. The same is true for us: When we come to the well, we meet Jesus and regain our hope and strength.

Anne Graham Lotz, the daughter of Billy and Ruth Graham, tells how she awakened early to spend time with the Lord while on vacation at the beach. Sitting on the porch, listening to the waves, she heard the Lord whisper, "Anne, what do you see?"

As she looked around, she answered:

Lord, I see little sandpipers running along the edge of
the water, making sure they keep out of reach of the
waves and don't get their feet wet. I see the skimmers
flying down the beach, just above the surf, skimming
the surface of the water with their long beaks. I see
seagulls standing in the tide up to their knees. And
then I see the pelicans who circle, then dive headfirst
into the waves, coming up with fish they seem to
swallow whole.[1]

Anne continued her story by describing what the Lord
seemed to say in return:

Anne, the Bible is like the ocean. And the people who
read My Word are very much like those birds. Some
will dance around the scriptures, not really wanting
to step in and get their feet wet in Bible study, but are
satisfied to just listen to their preacher or Bible teacher
tell them what the Bible says.

Others will read their Bibles, just skimming the
surface for facts and information. Some will get in
knee-deep, reading the Bible each day with a devotional or commentary close by for reference. And then
there are some like the pelicans, who dive in over their
heads, going deep in Bible study, applying and living
out what they learn. Which bird are you most like?[2]

Anne's challenge is our challenge. Which bird are we most
like? Or, in other words, how deep is our relationship with the
Lord? Do we invest time with Him or skim the surface?

Though our experience may differ from the woman at the
well in John 4, there comes a point in our life when we must

decide how wholeheartedly to embrace Jesus. He is the source of the living water we crave, and it's only through deep connection with Him that we will find the peace we seek. When we hit the proverbial brick wall, our pain (exemplified by the thirsty, weary, challenged, isolated woman at the well) meets hope (Jesus).

We often tie our desire for change to a special event or occasion. We focus on losing weight, getting in shape, changing our hairstyle, optimizing our skin care, getting a spray tan, practicing our makeup, or polishing our nails to be ready. Yet, our bridegroom, Jesus, invites us to be prepared now and always for our Christian walk (Matt. 25:1–13). We are running a continual, lifelong race. As such, we must prepare spiritually, emotionally, and physically for whatever the day may bring. So when we pause, come to the well, and focus on Him, we prepare ourselves for His work for today.

Many women I have spoken with regret their past decisions, actions, or lack of action as something that holds them back and keeps them from living freely in Him. One woman told me, "I try not to live in the past, but sometimes it is so easy to get swept away with all of my mistakes and things I wish I had done differently. When that happens, it is very hard to feel confident and take life by the reins."

Please lean into what I am saying next: We all make mistakes. We all have regrets. Accepting those is what allows us to move on and experience His freedom. Though there may be consequences from that part of our story, we can find our strength in Him. And we must pause and acknowledge the messages our inner critic repeatedly plays in our minds. When we become aware of those negative thoughts and verbalize them to God in prayer, we can surrender to Him and experience more of the abundant life He offers. It's okay when we mess up or fall short of the mark. Let's extend grace to ourselves and return to Him. Let's get back up and continue.

Seeing the Good in Our Lives

A couple of years ago, I was at the office working and seeing patients when we received a phone call from a woman traveling with the Imani Children's Choir. The choir consists of students from Uganda who travel to the US in small groups for three to six months. Based in Sebastian, Florida, they sing and raise funding and support around the US during their time abroad. Though the choir's members are orphans, they receive life necessities and an education.

One of the children, Paul, had developed a lesion on his skin, and their phone call was to ask me to look at it while they were passing through the area. Though I saw and treated Paul, getting to know him was the best gift.

While visiting with him in the exam room, I asked what surprised him the most about the US. Without hesitation, he said he was shocked at how many American children did not seem to appreciate or even like their educational opportunities. Routinely, the students would tell him, "I hate school." He was flabbergasted and saddened. He said, "They have buildings, AC, computers, supplies, books, homes, families, and endless opportunities to further their schooling. But they do not like it."

He couldn't help but compare the advantages that American children experienced to his own homeland's conditions.

"We start at 6 a.m. with our chores and have school from 7 a.m. to 6 p.m., with a two-hour break to prepare, eat, and clean up lunch. After dinner, students must clean the school. Then, we study until about 10 p.m."

Paul said he was getting up at 4 a.m. to get additional studying done and would sometimes stay up as late as midnight to provide more opportunities for success. In Uganda, children take a competitive test in eighth grade that determines if they can continue school or go straight to working for the rest of their lives. Another test in twelfth grade determines the same.

We—more specifically, my company—went on to adopt Paul financially. Nevertheless, our conversation left a lasting impression on how I view education.

After all, education equips us to fulfill God's purpose for creating us. Being open to learning and adapting will help us fill up on truth.

However, though the problem used to be access to information (the advent of the Gutenberg press turned that around as books became more readily available), today, the problem is often the accuracy of information. God calls you to—as Ronald Reagan said about his trusted advisors—"Trust but verify."[3] Let's avoid 24-hour news talk, which is meaningless when measured against the unwavering truth of God's Word. Though we can access information 24 hours a day, seven days a week through news talk, scrolling on our phones, and using the internet to look up anything we're interested in, should we? Studies have shown that the bombardment of this type of information negatively impacts our brains.[4] So, while education, reading, and learning are valuable for our lives, the source and volume of information must have boundaries placed on them for us to stay healthy. And our knowledge should always be measured by the only absolute truth, the Bible.

Perhaps even more importantly, my conversation with Paul reminded me of how often we fail to recognize the good in our lives. I love how John Mark Comer writes about how the things we pay attention to matter: "What we give our attention to is the person we become. The mind is the portal to the soul, and what we fill our minds with will shape the trajectory of our character."[5] The world's worries can crowd out all the good in our lives—family and friends, our purpose, and even our opportunity to experience an education. How can we trust Jesus and find our renewed hope in Him?

As we learn and understand this world, growing in His Word is crucial. The Bible is what gives our day-to-day life context and meaning. If Jesus is to be our source of strength, we must actively seek Him. We need His perspective on our day, challenges, fears, and relationships to thrive.

What is the one thing that seems to rock your world and rob you of peace most consistently? What triggers often serve as catalysts to make you feel like everything is up to you to accomplish on your own? What circumstances or situations cause you to tense up and become a control freak?

Asking these questions and journaling the answers will help you see when you are most vulnerable to fear and stress versus faith and resilience. These feelings are normal. There is nothing wrong with us feeling emotions. The choice comes when we must decide what to do with our feelings and how to grow beyond them. First, we can become aware of the small cues when they are happening. Only then can we change the default, leading us to the well—to Jesus.

My precious grandson is a young toddler. To say I am smitten with him is an understatement. I cherish every moment with him, both in person and on FaceTime. Grandparent love sends me over the moon! (And I have two more grandchildren on the way!)

However, in the last few months, he has started experiencing and expressing frustration and sadness. While these feelings are normal and part of our lives, we need to begin to learn a healthy way to communicate and deal with them at an early age. With that in mind, my husband and I have started helping him learn to breathe intentionally in and out to reset and be okay with the feeling. He got upset when he was at our home one day and wanted to play with something unsafe for him. I knelt so we were face-to-face and said, "I understand you are frustrated, and that is okay to feel. But this is not safe for you. So let's take a deep breath and blow it out three times." I then demonstrated what I meant.

During my first breath, he continued to fuss; with my second, he just looked at me with a curious, small smile; the third time, he almost laughed and then pursed his lips and blew air out with my last exhale. It was precious! But it took a reminder, a demonstration, and practice for him to begin incorporating that technique into his way of processing feelings. And it will take multiple reminders for him to choose that on his own.

While this may seem juvenile, we all need this kind of practice. Pausing, acknowledging what we are feeling, taking a few intentional breaths, and then visualizing Jesus at the well—waiting for us, speaking to us, leading and loving us—leads to peace and joy beyond our circumstances.

Come to the Well for Strength

When I feel most vulnerable, I try to think of God's way compared to the world's. I tell my patients that we are all about 60 percent water and must stay hydrated to function at our best. Our brain is 73 percent water, and function declines significantly with the slightest degree of dehydration. When we hydrate our bodies with water, every organ functions with greater strength and performance. [6] Spiritually, we are the same. Just as our bodies need water to maintain physical health, our spirits need the refreshment of the living water only Jesus can provide. When we approach the well of God's truth to obtain His living water, we gain the strength and vitality we need to go out into the world and serve Him.

Much more than merely revitalizing our spirits, the Bible's truths provide a guide to how we should live, a compass in the world, and protection from the enemy. The Bible compares our time spent in the Word as a way to combat the enemy's attacks on us. One of the best ways to do so is to don spiritual armor. In the first century, armor was protective and primarily defensive. In Ephesians 6:10–16 (NASB 1995), we read about the Armor of God.

After admonishing us to "Finally, be strong in the Lord and in the strength of His might" (verse 10), we are reminded of why we should do so: When we put on the whole armor of God, we have access to His strength. But we must first recognize our true enemy. As verse 12 says, "For our struggle is not against flesh and blood, but against the rulers, against the powers, against the world forces of this darkness, against the spiritual forces of wickedness in the heavenly places." Our struggle is not against other women, our spouse, friends, coworkers, or even "enemies" who have hurt us to the core. Though Satan may use them, they are not our actual opponents. Satan—our true enemy—is relentless, pacing like a lion who seeks to devour, distract, and rob us of our strength. This spiritual enemy never calls a truce.

Thankfully, wearing armor helps us "stand firm against the schemes of the devil." Because of the armor we wear, the power of God strengthens and upholds us. We need not fear the enemy or his schemes! As Elisha told his servant in 2 Kings 6:16 (NIV), "Do not fear, for those who are with us are more than those who are with them."

The lessons for us are significant when considering our health and well-being:

- Spiritually: The true Armor of God is needed because we will be wounded and knocked down every day by the world around us. We must armor up for the spiritual battle by staying close to Him.

- Emotionally: We can choose to let our hearts be protected from the emotional hurts of this world by allowing the Lord to touch and heal our wounds. When new insults come our way, we can combat them with His truths and live the abundant life He gives us.

- Physically: Do not let idleness or lack of proper nutrition and exercise weigh you down from God's promise of an abundant life of freedom and vitality. Choose Him by choosing to be a good steward of your body and mind in your daily choices.

To love God, we must know Him. What does it look like to seek to know anyone we love? We spend time with them. We lean in and listen to them, eager to truly see and understand who they are and what is important to them. Knowing Him gives us the strength we need to follow Him. ("But the people who know their God will display strength and take action" [Dan. 11:32 NASB 1995].)

We can spend time with God by reading His words, talking and praying to Him, and listening to His whispers and nudges. When we do, we will learn how to keep His commandments (John 14:15). God's love language is obedience. Yet we can only be obedient when we know Him; that, my beloved, takes time.

Corrie ten Boom once said, "If the devil can't make you sin, he'll make you busy."[7] Satan shows up throughout our days, but not as a cartoonish red person with two horns. No, he distracts us with text messages and alerts that invade our Bible time, with the desire to binge-watch television shows for too many hours, or with yet another committee or obligation. You and I can each name many things that take our time and minds away from God. Too easily, those things can become a distraction or even an idol in our lives.

I love the way John Ortberg talks about life's distractions. He said, "For many of us, the great danger is not that we will renounce our faith. It is that we will become so distracted and rushed and preoccupied that we will settle for a mediocre version of it. We will just skim our lives instead of actually living them."[8]

How disheartening! None of us wants to skim the surface of this life, never reaching deeper levels of truth or joy. Let's commit to seeking God more deeply, to approaching the well for spiritual nourishment. Each of us should come equipped with the desire to love Him more deeply and pursue the abundant life He has purposed and planned for us.

Facing Difficulties

On paper, Charles Krauthammer was enormously successful. Born in New York City and raised in Montreal, Krauthammer was educated at McGill University (BA 1970), Oxford University (Commonwealth Scholar in Politics) and Harvard (MD 1975). While serving as chief resident in psychiatry at the Massachusetts General Hospital, he co-discovered a form of bipolar disease.

Then, in 1978, he quit his medical practice and came to Washington to help direct planning in psychiatric research in the Carter administration. In 1980, he served as a speechwriter to Vice President Walter Mondale. He then became a Fox News commentator.

Despite his professional success, Krauthammer's life was challenging. He went from being a twenty-three-year-old medical student one day to a person with paraplegia the next after a medical school pool party and diving accident. But he went on to accomplish much due to a remarkable ability to accept his new reality.

Charles Krauthammer's response is one that we can learn from, too. All too often, we must embrace our reality, accepting both the good and bad, the obstacles and the challenges. Life's difficulties can derail us if we are not prepared to embrace what is and surrender our lives fully to Him in acceptance.

The truth is that God is continually molding us, especially with the trials and difficulties we experience. Let's consider the example described in 1 Peter. Written in 64 AD from Rome (symbolic Babylon), the epistle presents Christ as the believer's example and source of hope in times of suffering in a spiritually hostile world. In it, Peter tells believers that persecution can lead to growth (*Wow!*) or bitterness (*Ow!*). It's our response that determines the result.

When we experience challenges at school, work, or home, we must accept our current circumstances and recognize what we cannot change. In return, some of those difficulties will prove invaluable because they can help perfect us. As 1 Peter 5:10 (ESV) notes, "After you have suffered for a little while, the God of all grace, who called you to his eternal glory in Christ, will himself restore, confirm, strengthen and establish you." The divine perspective of suffering is to endure without wavering in our faith. Yet doing so often proves difficult because we must relinquish our tight grip on control.

Acceptance is powerful because it frees us from trying to control our circumstances and gives us relief through trusting all things to God. Many of us have heard the Serenity Prayer, a common name for a prayer written by American theologian Reinhold Niebuhr (1892–1971). The best-known form is "God, grant me the serenity to accept the things I cannot change, courage to change the things I can, and wisdom to know the difference."

In this instance, wisdom comes from knowing when to accept certain truths and when to challenge them. But our acceptance should not be considered a weakness. After all, in Luke 1:38, we are told that Mary accepted the angel's words regarding her pregnancy: "And Mary said, 'Behold the bond-slave of the Lord; may it be done to me according to your word.' And the angel departed her." Far from demonstrating weakness, Mary's acceptance was a powerful declaration of faith.

Whenever I feel sorry for myself or argue about my current circumstances, I remember how my tight grip on control isn't as powerful as I think it is anyway. I remember the words God spoke as he challenged Job in his way of thinking:

> Where were you when I laid the foundation of the
> earth? Tell Me, if you have understanding, who set its

measurements? Since you know. Or who stretched the line on it? On what were its bases sunk? Or who laid its cornerstone, when the morning stars sang together and all the sons of God shouted for joy? Or who enclosed the sea with doors, when it went out from the womb, bursting forth; When I made a cloud its garment, and thick darkness its swaddling bands, and I placed boundaries on it And I set a bolt and doors, and I said, "Thus far you shall come, but no farther; and here shall your proud waves stop?" (Job 38:4–11 NASB 1995)

You and I can only see a small part of the big picture, but God sees it all. Our limited understanding can never offer the same level of comfort we have in knowing that God sees the full scope of this world. What a comfort there is in knowing that no challenge we face will ever surprise Him! He is unfazed by every difficulty we will ever encounter, and because of His great love for us, we are always better served by trusting in Him than by attempting to walk the path of life alone. Exodus 13:17, which describes the challenges the Israelites faced after leaving Egypt and God's response to them, reminds us of this truth: "Now when Pharaoh had let the people go, God did not lead them by the way of the land of the Philistines, even though it was near; for God said, 'The people might change their minds when they see war and return to Egypt.'"

God may take us on the long way, but it's always the right way. And according to Oswald Chambers, when we know and trust in Him, we can rest assured that "Faith is deliberate confidence in the character of God whose ways you may not understand at the time."[9]

As we close this chapter, I invite you to sit in a comfortable position and close your eyes. Imagine an endless well of water with reflections of the sun dancing along the tiny ripples of movement. Think of Jesus as the source of living water that quenches our thirsty souls and the light of our lives that permeates all aspects of our spirit. Remind yourself that He never leaves us and is always there, beckoning us to come to Him. We may need renewed strength, a deeper acceptance of our present circumstances, a new hope and purpose, or healing for the wounds in our hearts. Whatever we need can be found in Him. Before opening your eyes and continuing your day, commit to incorporating practices that remind you to come to His well daily. Just as the woman at the well (John 4) was forever changed, you will be too.

SNAP

Seek Him

A few moments with Jesus can transform us. When we come to the well, we meet Jesus and regain our hope and strength.

MEDITATE ON THESE WORDS

✟ It was for freedom that Christ set us free; therefore keep standing firm and do not be subject again to a yoke of slavery. (Gal. 5:1)

✟ For you were called to freedom, brethren; only do not turn your freedom into an opportunity for the flesh, but through love serve one another. (Gal. 5:13)

✟ [F]or he who has died is freed from sin. (Rom. 6:7)

✟ Owe nothing to anyone except to love one another; for he who loves his neighbor has fulfilled the law. (Rom. 13:8)

✟ Now the Lord is the Spirit, and where the Spirit of the Lord is, there is liberty. (2 Cor. 3:17)

✟ [A]nd you will know the truth, and the truth will make you free. (John 8:32)

✠ Act as free men, and do not use your freedom as a covering for evil, but use it as bondslaves of God. Honor all people, love the brotherhood, fear God, honor the king. (1 Pet. 2:16–17)

✠ From my distress I called upon the LORD; The LORD answered me and set me in a large place. (Ps. 118:5)

✠ The Spirit of the Lord GOD is upon me, because the LORD has anointed me to bring good news to the afflicted; He has sent me to bind up the brokenhearted, to proclaim liberty to captives and freedom to prisoners. (Isa. 61:1)

✠ So if the Son makes you free, you will be free indeed. (John 8:36)

✠ [A]nd having been freed from sin, you became slaves of righteousness. (Rom. 6:18)

✠ For the law of the Spirit of life in Christ Jesus has set you free from the law of sin and of death. (Rom. 8:2)

Nourish Self

Focus on approaching the well for nourishment in two ways:

1. Physical Thirst: Set a goal to drink more water and adequately hydrate every organ in your body. Our bodies need pure water daily, but drinking that does not factor into the American consumerism equation well. Many advertisements try to persuade us that we

must have flavors, artificial and chemical sweeteners, or other substances to enjoy our drinks. However, do not buy into this belief. Instead, save money and save your health.

- A good measure is half your body weight in ounces (so if someone weighs 150 pounds, they should aim for 75 ounces of water).
- Drink plain water, although adding a slice of orange, lime, or lemon is okay.
- How do you know if you've had enough water? Your urine should be clear.

2. Spiritual Thirst: We are easily worn down and tired from this world's noise, chaos, disappointments, and fears. Commit to spending time at the well.

- Set up a time and date with Jesus every day— whether that's ten minutes or an hour. Put it on your calendar.
- Whatever season you are in, find a method that allows you to hear truth and hope every day. Ideas include listening to podcasts, books, or sermons; reading the Word; using a devotional for guidance; getting a daily Bible that is chronological for morning or evening; journaling your prayers; or attending weekly services and classes at your local church.

Armor of God

As we read Ephesians 6:10–18, the first three aspects of the armor are things we clothe ourselves in (gird your loins with truth, put on the breastplate of righteousness, shod your feet with the gospel of peace). The next three are items we actively pick up (the shield of faith, the helmet of salvation, and the sword of the Spirit—the Word of God).

For this chapter, let's focus on the last two aspects of armor. Set your mind on your salvation. Cover your thoughts daily—just as you would place a helmet on your head—with a focus on our true home, Heaven. Then, pick up the Word of God, your road map to your real home. When you do, you'll experience the living water of Jesus and the well of love, grace, and mercy He provides.

Prayer

DEAR HEAVENLY FATHER,

WE PRAISE YOU FOR YOUR WILLINGNESS TO MEET US AT the well. We are humbled by Your offering of the true water of life found in the truths of Your Word.

Help us to pause daily and reflect on what You tell us about dealing with our sadness and frustrations. Guide us to accept what is and trust You with the details of what we do not understand. Allow us to place at Your feet anything holding us back from the life You have offered us.

We seek Your face as we navigate and strive to set ourselves apart from the worries and cares of this world. We trust You. We rely on You. We desire to see and know You in a new way today as we move more freely after spending time with You!

In Jesus's name,

Amen.

CHAPTER 10

You've Got This

*A*s I was getting ready to leave the house recently, I heard a comment on the television that prompted me to pause and listen. *Merriam-Webster* had announced the word of the year was "authentic."[1] Reading about it later, I was struck by the commentary on how, with the increasing ability of technology to manipulate images or create deep fakes, it can be hard to tell what's real from what's fake. We can't always trust what we see.

"Authentic" is defined in several ways, including "not false or imitation," "true to one's own personality, spirit, or character," and "made or done the same way as an original," among others.[2] In describing "authentic" as the word of the year, *Merriam-Webster* commented, "Although clearly a desirable quality, 'authentic' is hard to define and subject to debate—two reasons it sends many people to the dictionary."[3]

I smiled in appreciation of the importance of such a word. In a world that is progressing rapidly to use technology to skew reality in the pursuit of supposed perfection, we are still drawn to what is genuine. And that is what God calls us to do, as well. He invites us to show up as our beautiful, authentic selves daily. You, my friend, are special, loved, and worthy. You do not need to be anyone other than who God has called you to be.

Authentic beauty embraces all the parts of ourselves. For instance, I'm an introvert who adores people. I love football and basketball but do not enjoy shopping. I'm all about communication but dislike talking on the phone. I'm grounded in faith but fascinated by science and medicine. I embrace getting sweaty riding my bike but wear makeup to yoga; I choose comfy clothes when running errands but love to dress up for dates. I love to garden but struggle to keep plants alive. I'm a visual learner but not an artist, I love horses but fear cats, and I enjoy being social but don't like social media. Those are all parts of myself that I've chosen to accept—even if they don't fit the world's definition of who or what I should be. We need not feel boxed in by stereotypes or feel we need to fulfill expectations when the truth is that we are loved and accepted by God, just as we are.

As Judy Garland once said, "Be the first-rate version of yourself and not the second-rate version of somebody else."[4] The message here is twofold. We can take the time to explore who we are and use that self-awareness to help us live authentically. It can be tempting to compare our lives with other people's lives. But as we shift from a horizontal focus (comparing ourselves to others) to a vertical focus (focusing on our relationship with Jesus), we go from feeling lost and discouraged to finding hope, rest, and freedom.

When we focus less on what those around us are doing and more on serving Jesus, we often find contentment with our lives. A woman in her fifties once told me that as she reflects on the past twenty years, she has learned lessons she wishes her younger self knew: "Even though I have more wrinkles, my life is complicated, and my joints hurt more, I try to take the time and energy to look for the resources and people that can help me deal with the hard things in life so that I can serve the Lord well until my last breath," she said. "Looking back, I'd love to tell my thirty-year-old self these truths."

Time is precious, and each of us has the privilege of fulfilling our God-given purpose while we're here on earth. That knowledge can motivate, but it also imbues us with a sense of responsibility. As Robert Moffat once noted, "We have all eternity to celebrate our victories, but only one short hour before sunset in which to win them."[5] How will we use the time we have available to us?

Armor and Prayer

In chapter 9, we discussed the purpose of spiritual armor in thwarting the enemy's schemes. But the truth is that this practice has much more profound, eternal implications: When we claim our authentic beauty and clothe ourselves with spiritual armor, we are ready to move forward and fulfill the God-given purpose of our lives.

Spiritual armor provides the daily equipment we need to equip and allow us to do the job God has called us to. In Ephesians 6:13–18 (NIV), the author reminds us of the importance of doing so:

> Therefore put on the full armor of God, so that when the day of evil comes, you may be able to stand your ground, and after you have done everything, to stand. Stand firm then, with the belt of truth buckled around your waist, with the breastplate of righteousness in place, and with your feet fitted with the readiness that comes from the gospel of peace. In addition to all this, take up the shield of faith, with which you can

extinguish all the flaming arrows of the evil one. Take the helmet of salvation and the sword of the Spirit, which is the word of God. And pray in the Spirit on all occasions with all kinds of prayers and requests. With this in mind, be alert and always keep on praying for all the Lord's people.

Verse 14 reminds us to begin with the belt of truth buckled around our waist. When we do, we avoid the deceitfulness and moral relativism of the world and focus on God's truth. Next, we need to don the breastplate of righteousness. It should not go unnoticed that righteousness begins in our hearts (Prov. 4:23).

After that, we must ensure our feet are shod with the gospel of peace. When we walk in peace, worry and anxiety may still be present in our lives, but we can take comfort in knowing that He equips us with tools to help combat them. Did you know that we are the most medicated society in the history of the world?[6] Medication has its place and can be highly effective, but I wonder if one of the reasons we turn to it is the need for more peace. Our world is stressful, anxiety-inducing, and rapidly changing, and it bombards us with division, strife, and danger. Many numb themselves with alcohol, drugs, work, or addictions of all kinds to cope.

On its own, this world has no peace, but this shouldn't come as a surprise. After all, the Bible says that we will have trouble in this world, but the good news is that Jesus promised to give us peace that surpasses all understanding. Without God, we are not equipped to manage anxiety and fear.

Interestingly, the Bible is the most highlighted book on Kindle.[7] Even more compelling, the most highlighted passage is Philippians 4:6–7 (NASB 1995): "Be anxious for nothing, but in everything by prayer and supplication with thanksgiving let your requests be made known to God. And the peace of God, which surpasses all comprehension, will guard your hearts and minds in Christ Jesus."

As Christians, we will feel anxious and fearful at times; those emotions are real. But we need not become prisoners to them. Instead, we are to walk in His peace.

We look to Him to grant us the strength and peace to walk in His ways. But what does it look like to arm ourselves in the way Ephesians describes?

There is a running joke in our family that I make sound effects when emphasizing a point. And I have to be very careful not to do that when speaking. It stems from riding horses for years; that is how I communicated with them. But on extra difficult days, I like to pretend I am cinching down my armor extra tight and make the sound effect for putting armor on.

Then, we pick up our shield of faith. We must work continually to grow our faith. We can never reach the point where we believe we know or have total faith. Instead, we must stay humble and willing to read and study with an open heart and mind.

Next, we can strap on the helmet of salvation. Believing in the saving power of Jesus can transform our minds from focusing solely on this world to knowing that Heaven is our true home.

Then, we must focus on the sword of the spirit—in other words, we must read, meditate, and memorize the Word of God.

We should utilize whatever it takes to go into the world with courage and no fear. As Ephesians 2:10 reminds us, "For we are His workmanship, created in Christ Jesus for good works, which God prepared beforehand so that we would walk in them." God has already prepared the work. It's ready for us.

In the final verse describing spiritual armor, the author reminds readers that prayer is essential: "And pray in the Spirit on all occasions with all kinds of prayers and requests. With this in mind, be alert and always keep on praying for all the Lord's people" (Eph. 6:18 NIV).

Praying at all times and in the Spirit is what activates our armor.

Several years ago, I spent a year studying prayer. I began a new dialogue of talking to God all day, verbally and in my head. I made a "war room" in my closet. I started journaling my prayers and answers to my prayers. And over time, it became a powerful exercise for me to look back and see all the ways God had walked with me and answered my prayers.

Prayer confirms our dependence on Him because there are also many unanswered—or at least seemingly unanswered—prayers.

It also leads to tranquility. As 1 Timothy 2:1–2 (NASB 1995) reminds us, "I urge that entreaties and prayers, petitions and thanksgivings, be made on behalf of all men, for kings and all who are in authority, so that we may lead a tranquil and quiet life in all godliness and dignity."

Yet many of us struggle to make prayer a regular part of our faith. Some of it stems from the fact that we aren't sure what to pray about, but reframing our vision of prayer can help alter our perspective. As Mother Teresa said, "I am not called to be successful; I am called to be faithful."[8]

Over time, I've come to use this loose framework in my approach to prayer:

1. Start with acknowledging and praising God for His sovereign presence, provision, and grace!

2. Pray for myself. Tell the Lord what is on my heart and mind that is creating worry or fear. Ask for specific requests or concerns. Ask for acceptance of the hard things. Ask for direction with the unknowns. Ask for courage and discipline to steward my health and life choices in a way that honors Him.

3. Pray for others. As we pray for others, we affirm the unfolding good in their lives. We could even pray for those who have harmed us, because it is difficult not to have compassion for those we are lifting to God. As Jesus reminds us in Matthew 5:44 (NIV), "But I tell you, love your enemies and pray for those who persecute you."

4. Pray while believing because doing so is powerful and effective. James 5:16 says, "The prayer of a righteous person is powerful and effective." When we are faithful to God in our intercession, we fight our battles on our knees and trust Him. He hears, and He certainly answers.

5. Pray in His will. Jesus demonstrates this concept in the Garden of Gethsemane: "And He said, 'Abba, Father, all things are possible for You. Take this cup away from Me; nevertheless, not what I will, but what You will'" (Mark 14:36 NKJV). As Gary Henry reminds us in *Diligently Seeking God*, "Rather than come to God with a demanding spirit, we should pray with a buoyant trust, grateful that we can put ourselves

in His hands. It can be a delight to let Him decide what is best."⁹ But when we pray, it is helpful to pray with what might be called a "listening" attitude. As we make our supplications to God, we are to be open to the possibility that He may have a better plan or higher purpose.

Praying for God's will to be done can be an agonizing experience, without question. It was so for our Lord in Gethsemane. And yet, an agonizing experience is not necessarily negative in the long run. To let God choose which path we are to follow is, at least for us, to grow in our spirits. It is, as Ralph Washington Sockman said, to be made more wise: "To pray is to expose the shores of the mind to the incoming tide of God."¹⁰

Let's deepen our prayer lives for His wisdom, discernment, direction, provision, belonging, and comfort. When we do, we will find the peace we seek no matter our circumstances: "You keep him in perfect peace whose mind is stayed on You, because he trusts in You. Trust in the Lord forever, for the Lord God is an everlasting rock" (Isa. 26:3–4 ESV).

Using Our One, Precious Life

One year, the church invited my grandmother Biggs to be one of twelve models for a calendar they were putting together to highlight the congregation's widows. The church hired hair stylists, make-up artists, clothing stylists, and a photographer for the shoot. On the day of the photoshoot, my grandmother found out that she would be Ms. January. She came alive!

After the morning shoot, Grandmother Biggs visited my home and radiated joy. She looked beautiful and felt beautiful.

Those twelve women—including my grandmother—felt seen and appreciated that day. One of them even said that when the stylist met her that morning with a hug, she felt profoundly grateful because she hadn't been hugged since her husband had passed away two years earlier. The simple gesture of a hug gave her joy. Those ladies felt purpose, and, more importantly, they felt a connection that day.

Seeing each other in person, touching each other in a friendly, kind way, and giving life to others feeds our souls and improves our health and well-being. Throughout scripture, Jesus tells people's stories. He spoke of times when he was with them, how he connected eye-to-eye with others, and how those relationships were fruitful, powerful, and necessary. We cannot be with Jesus physically now, but His presence is known through the written Word of the Bible and felt through His Holy Spirit, giving us the ability to know Him.

We are made for social connection, and there are multiple ways we can connect with people, know them, and gain joy and wisdom from them while we also receive the opportunity to be known. This connection can occur through time spent in person, over the phone, through FaceTime or Zoom, via a personal written note, or by reading a book or the written word. Yet how we "show up" for those connections combined with our motivation for what we put out there through social media determines if that connection is life-giving and authentic or chasing the need to feel a void of loneliness, isolation, or low self-worth/purpose.

Donning our spiritual armor and praying wholeheartedly are necessary for us to speak and fulfill the Great Commission boldly. But they are also essential for us to make the connections with others that God has asked of us. We must be ready and obedient to go anywhere God asks. It could be across the street, to the next desk at work, or overseas, where Christians face persecution. Perhaps it's simply the request to give up some leisure or entertainment time a few nights a week for meet-ups and Bible studies. (Hebrews 10:25 calls us to encourage one another to love and good deeds.)

Those Christ-led connections can arise in the most unlikely places. I'm reminded of the end of the Esther Event we held at work. Just as we were saying our goodbyes, a woman in her early eighties stopped me. She thanked me for a wonderful day and then told me that she had never really read the Bible. Growing up, her family owned a large Bible that sat on the coffee table, but no one read it or talked about it.

"I had no idea there was so much to the Bible," she said. She then mentioned that she lived about an hour away but continued to say: "I am not driving home without stopping first to buy myself a Bible. Thank you."

With that, she turned and left with a determined step.

As thoughts flooded my brain, I was paralyzed with gratitude. *Praise you, Lord, for the gift of Your Word. Thank you for allowing this lady to see You through the events of this day.*

I felt overwhelming gratitude that I had been encouraged to read the Bible from a young age. I also felt more empowered than ever before to stop assuming others know the Lord and speak more boldly of the beauty of who He is.

Friends, when we fulfill the Great Commission, we declare the goodness of God. As Psalm 71:18 (NASB 1995) reminds us, "And even when I am old and gray, O God, do not forsake me, until I declare Your strength to this generation, your power to all who are to come." This lifelong journey does not end. The book of 2 Timothy was written near the end of Paul's life, and he sounds worn out, weary, and tired. Yet even then, he admonishes us to focus on being able to utter the words, "I have fought the good fight, I have finished the course, I have kept the faith" (2 Tim. 4:7).

Recently, I was called into a patient's room. She had noted a lesion on her skin and wanted me to examine the area. During our conversation, she told me she was moving to a new city and returning to school after a difficult time in her life.

"Wow!" I said. "You've got this. You go, girl!" (The phrase "you go, girl" is used to encourage and celebrate women's achievements, strength, and capability. It's a rallying cry.[11])

In response, the woman immediately started weeping and laughing at the same time. In her fifties, she was living out a bold belief in herself but still appreciated my encouragement. We all want to see others believe in us, cheer for us, and see us for who we truly are. Choose to be the cheerleader and encourager, knowing it does not detract from your value.

What will we make of this one precious life we have received?

I believe it's possible for everyone who picks up this book to find and live out a bold belief in themselves. When we delight in our choices and surrender to the provision of God, He will transform our mind, body, and soul to reveal the beauty we possess. Let's love the journey, embrace the challenges, make healthy choices, and live out our authentic beauty.

S N A P

Seek Him

I encourage you to claim your authentic beauty! Clothe yourselves with the spiritual armor God offers and fulfill the God-given purpose of your life!

MEDITATE ON THESE WORDS

✝ For this God is our God for ever and ever; he will be our guide even to the end. (Ps. 48:14 NIV)

✝ Be very careful, then, how you live—not as unwise but as wise, making the most of every opportunity, because the days are evil. (Eph. 5:15–16)

✝ I planted the seed, Apollos watered it, but God has been making it grow. So neither the one who plants nor the one who waters is anything, but only God, who makes things grow. The one who plants and the one who waters have one purpose, and they will each be rewarded according to their own labor. (1 Cor. 3:6–8)

✝ To all in Rome who are loved by God and called to be his holy people: Grace and peace to you from God our Father and from the Lord Jesus Christ. . . . If we live, we live for the Lord; and if we die, we die for the

Lord. So, whether we live or die, we belong to the Lord. (Rom. 1:7, 14:8)

✝ I have been crucified with Christ and I no longer live, but Christ lives in me. The life I now live in the body, I live by faith in the Son of God, who loved me and gave himself for me. (Gal. 2:20)

✝ Since we live by the Spirit, let us keep in step with the Spirit. (Gal. 5:25)

✝ This is what the LORD says to Israel: "Seek me and live; . . . Seek good, not evil, that you may live. Then the LORD God Almighty will be with you, just as you say he is." (Amos 5:4; 5:14)

✝ Because your love is better than life, my lips will glorify you. I will praise you as long as I live, and in your name I will lift up my hands. (Ps. 63:3–4)

✝ I will sing to the LORD all my life; I will sing praise to my God as long as I live. (Ps. 104:33)

✝ Live as free people, but do not use your freedom as a cover-up for evil; live as God's slaves. (1 Pet. 2:16)

✝ For we live by faith, not by sight. (2 Cor. 5:7)

Nourish Self

Activity 1: Ponder some of these quotes.

- "I want to be all used up when this life is over" (Anonymous).

- "There needs to be a healthy sense of urgency in our lives," says Gary Henry. "With regard to that which the Lord wants us to do in His work individually, there is not an unlimited amount of time in which to do that work. Each of us has a 'window of opportunity,' and after that is gone, we will give account for our stewardship of the time given us. We urgently need to 'redeem the time,' as Paul put it."[12]

- "There's no prerequisites to worthiness," says Viola Davis. "You're born worthy . . ."[13]

Now, remind yourself that you are the loved, adored, cherished daughter of God. He is with you every step of the way in this life, through all of the twists, turns, disappointments, roadblocks, detours, and fears. He guides you as you follow.

So go about your day unshackled, free, and with great joy and confidence.

Activity 2: Develop a practice of daily prayer.

1. Make prayer a part of your breathing, a constant companion. As 1 Thessalonians 5:17 reminds us, "Pray without ceasing."

2. Shut off your device or other distractions and start. Now is the best time to begin.

3. Talk to Him and, most importantly, be still to listen to Him. Be so familiar with God that it is as though He is audibly speaking to you. Listen for His nudges and whispers. See Psalm 46:10: "Be still and know that I am God."

4. Write down your prayers. Journal them. (Shred them if you want.) It's not a literary piece; it's from your heart. Or utilize a prayer journal that is beautiful and helpful, like the *Rhythms Prayer Journal* from Val Marie Paper.

5. Look back and see all God has done with you, through you, and for you. He is always ahead of us.

Armor of God

In his book *Every Day in His Presence*, Charles F. Stanley reminds readers that whenever they feel inadequate to serve God, they should remember that he isn't looking for perfection. Instead, what He actually requires is sensitivity to the Spirit (attentive to promptings), service (serving others rather than self), sacrifice (pouring self out for Him), self-denial (seeking His goals, not your own), and suffering (following Him no matter the cost). As Stanley reflects, "In other words, the Savior wants to use your life as a platform for His power. So when He calls, don't worry about whether you're smart, talented, or beautiful enough. Just obey Him wholeheartedly. He will surely magnify Himself through you."[14]

How can concentrating on what God requires of us refocus our attention on Him and off of ourselves? How does that inform the way we live?

Prayer

DEAR HEAVENLY FATHER,

$\mathcal{A}$S WE PAUSE TO PRAISE YOU AT THE END OF THIS journey, equip us to be our authentic selves. Guide us to see what You see in us. Allow us to embrace ourselves as we are, even as we strive to grow in our understanding and knowledge of You continually; in our stewardship of our physical, mental, and emotional health; and in surrendering our lives to You.

Guide our choices daily as we work to live out of our desire to honor and glorify You with every decision.

Then, help us to see others in our path—the ones You place there—as opportunities to talk about You and Your relentless and unending love for all.

Help us to speak hope and truth throughout this precious life that You have blessed us with, even as we keep our hearts and minds fixed on our real home, Heaven.

In Jesus's name,

Amen.

Evelyn M. Jones

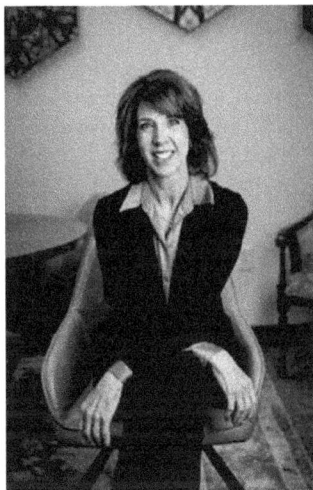

EVELYN M. JONES is the founder of WellSprings Institute and the EMJ product line. Dr. Jones has more than thirty years of experience as a board-certified dermatologist practicing general, surgical, and cosmetic dermatology. She is passionate about the preventative side of medicine and regularly speaks on spiritual and physical wellness to women of all ages. She strives to empower people to make healthy lifestyle choices with a goal to augment skin health, prevent chronic disease, and improve overall health.

Dr. Jones believes all women can reclaim their God-given beauty despite all of the wounding, hurt, and inner and outer voices that speak to the contrary. She believes in the power of knowing we are enough, chosen, and deeply loved. Dr. Jones is passionate about walking alongside women of all ages to educate and empower them to claim their authentic beauty and honor God in healthy choices.

NOTES

Chapter 1

1   Mother Teresa, in Richard Innes and Crystal B., "Called to Be Faithful," ACTS International, accessed February 8, 2024, https://www.actsweb. org/articles/article.php?i=2597&d=2&c=2.

Chapter 2

1   Anne Lamott (@AnneLamottQuote), "'No" is a complete sentence. It's given me this tremendous sense of power. I'm a little bit drunk on it," Twitter (now X), October 18, 2017, 8:27 a.m., https://twitter.com/ AnneLamottQuote/status/920657616707182592?lang=en.

2   Design Your Life with Dennis and Thammie Sy, "Busy Is the New Stupid by Bill Gates and Warren Buffett," YouTube Video, 1:34, accessed November 16, 2023, https://www.youtube.com/ watch?v=qsjET4AClyo.

Chapter 3

1   Daniel P. Miller, Jane Waldfogel, and Wen-Jui Han, "Family Meals and Child Academic and Behavioral Outcomes," *Child Development* 83, no. 6 (August 7, 2012): 2104–2120, https://doi.org/10.1111/j.1467 8624.2012.01825.x.

2   Sheri Rose Shepherd, *His Princess Every Day Devotional: Love Letters from Your King* (Washington, DC: Salem Books, 2019), Kindle.

3   Christa Black, *God Loves Ugly: & love makes beautiful,* reprint ed. (Nashville: FaithWords, 2013), Kindle.

4   Hippocrates, *The Aphorisms of Hippocrates* (New York: Collins, 1817), n.p.

5   Zonya Foco, "How Many Servings of Fruit & Vegetables Do You Eat, Really? Zonya, accessed February 8, 2024, https://zonya.com/articles/ how-many-servings-fruits-vegetables-do-you-really-eat/.

6   Kelsey Kloss, "139 Nutrition Statistics You Need to Know," Livestrong, updated December 22, 2023, https://www.livestrong.com/ article/13731066-nutrition-statistics/.

7   Roni Caryn Rabin, "What Foods Are Banned in Europe but Not Banned in the US?" *The New York Times,* Well | Eat, December 28, 2018, https://www.nytimes.com/2018/12/28/well/eat/food-additives-banned-europe-united-states.html.

8   Chartwell, "9 Lessons on Health and Longevity from the World's Blue Zones," 2023, https://chartwell.com/en/blog/2018/02/9-lessons-on-health-and-longevity-from-the-world%E2%80%99s-blue-zones.

Chapter 4

1   Chartwell, "9 Lessons."

2   Katrina L. Piercy, Richard P. Troiano, Rachel M. Ballard, Susan A. Carlson, Janet E. Fulton, Deborah A. Galuska, Stephanie M. George, and Richard D. Olson, "The Physical Activity Guidelines for Americans," *JAMA* 320, no. 19 (November 20, 2018): 2020–28, https://doi.org/10.1001/jama.2018.14854.

3   Office of Disease Prevention and Health Promotion, "Current Guidelines | Health.gov," August 24, 2021, https://health.gov/our-work/nutrition-physical-activity/physical-activity-guidelines/current-guidelines.

4   Betsy Mikel, "1 Simple Way to Help Kids Perform Better at School (It Works for Adults, Too), *Inc.*, March 23, 2017, https://www.inc.com/betsy-mikel/science-says-kids-learn-better-when-their-teachers-do-this.html#:~:text=Moving%20more%20helps%20make%20you,is%20great%20for%20your%20brain.

Chapter 5

1   Centers for Disease Control and Prevention, "Adolescent and School Health | CDC," September 4, 2020, https://www.cdc.gov/healthyyouth/.

2   Alexa Mikhail, "Loneliness Is a Public Health Crisis, Comparable to Smoking up to 15 Cigarettes a Day," *Fortune* | Well, June 15, 2023, https://fortune.com/well/2023/06/15/loneliness-comparable-to-smoking-up-to-15-cigarettes-a-day/.

3   Mikhail, "Loneliness," *Fortune.*

4   Regis College, "Does Social Media Create Isolation?" Regis College Online, December 23, 2019, https://online.regiscollege.edu/blog/does-social-media-create-isolation/.

5   Genesis Games, "The Impact of Social Media on Relationships," The Gottman Institute, February 10, 2022, https://www.gottman.com/blog/the-impact-of-social-media-on-relationships/.

6   Games, "Social Media on Relationships," The Gottman Institute.

7   Jacq Spence, "Nonverbal Communication: How Body Language & Nonverbal Cues Are Key," Lifesize, February 18, 2020, https://www.lifesize.com/blog/speaking-without-words/.

8   Albert Mehrabian, *Silent Messages* (Belmont, CA: Wadsworth, 1972), 76–77.

9   Rob Brockman, "5 Biblical Principles for Social Media," The Gospel Coalition | Canada, September 27, 2021, https://ca.thegospelcoalition.org/article/5-biblical-principles-for-social-media/.

10 Brockman, "Biblical Principles," The Gospel Coalition | Canada.

11 Dan Buettner, *The Blue Zones Solution: Eating and Living Like the World's Healthiest People* (Washington, DC: National Geographic, 2015), Kindle.

12 Buettner, *Blue Zones Solution,* Kindle.

13 Buettner, *Blue Zones Solution,* Kindle.

14 Sarina Schrager, "Integrating Behavioral Health into Primary Care," *Farm Practice Management* 28, no. 3 (June 1, 2021):3–4.

15 Mayo Clinic, "Chronic Stress Puts Your Health at Risk," Mayo Foundation for Medical Education and Research, July 8, 2021, https://www.mayoclinic.org/healthy-lifestyle/stress-management/in-depth/stress/art-20046037.

16 Mayo Clinic, "Chronic Stress."

17 Boyd Bailey, "Be Still," Wisdom Hunters, July 28, 2021, https://www.wisdomhunters.com/be-still-2/.

18 Lamott (@AnneLamottQuote), "'No' is a complete sentence. . . ." Twitter.

19 Hunt Allcott et al., "Welfare Effects," *American Economic Review.*

20 Olivia Solon, "Ex-Facebook President Sean Parker: Site Made to Exploit Human 'Vulnerability,'" *The Guardian*, November 9, 2017, https://www.theguardian.com/technology/2017/nov/09/facebook-sean-parker-vulnerability-brain-psychology.

21 Patrick Nelson, "We Touch Our Phones 2,617 Times a Day," July 7, 2016, Networkworld, https://www.networkworld.com/article/953059/we-touch-our-phones-2617-times-a-day-says-study.html.

Chapter 6

1   *The Oprah Winfrey Show,* season 23, episode 82, "What Can You Live Without Experiment (Pt. 2)," aired March 2, 2009, Amanda Cash, producer, CBS Television Distribution, 2009, https://www.youtube.com/watch?v=Y7gk4Ur7-EE.

2   Joshua Becker, "Don't Just Declutter, De-own," in *Becoming Minimalist* (podcast), 4:28, November 19, 2021, https://www.youtube.com/watch?v=-faHfZOdFiY.

3 Emily Freeman, *The Next Right Thing: A Simple, Soulful Practice for Making Life Decisions* (Ada, MI: Revell, 2019), Kindle.

4 C. S. Lewis, *Mere Christianity* (New York: Touchstone, 1996), 87–88.

5 Don Colbert, *Deadly Emotions: Understand the Mind-Body-Spirit Connection that Can Heal or Destroy You* (Nashville: Thomas Nelson, 2020), Kindle.

6 Colbert, *Deadly Emotions,* Kindle.

7 Colbert, *Deadly Emotions,* Kindle.

Chapter 7

1 Skin Cancer Foundation, "Skin Cancer Facts & Statistics: What You Need to Know," updated February 2024, https://www.skincancer.org/skin-cancer-information/skin-cancer-facts/#:~:text=About%2090%20percent%20of%20nonmelanoma,UV)%20radiation%20from%20the%20sun.&text=Basal%20cell%20carcinoma%20(BCC)%20-is,in%20the%20U.S.%20each%20year.

2 "Sunscreen and Your Morning Routine," Johns Hopkins Medicine | Health, accessed January 29, 2024, https://www.hopkinsmedicine.org/health/wellness-and-prevention/sunscreen-and-your-morning-routine.

3 National Institutes of Health, "Vitamin D Fact Sheet for Professionals," updated September 18, 2023, https://ods.od.nih.gov/factsheets/VitaminD-HealthProfessional/.

4 Harvard Health Publishing, Harvard Medical School, "Time for More Vitamin D," September 1, 2008, https://www.health.harvard.edu/staying-healthy/time-for-more-vitamin-d.

5 National Academies, "Sunscreen Does Not Cause Vitamin D Deficiency," March 31, 2019, https://www.nationalacademies.org/based-on-science/sunscreen-does-not-cause-vitamin-d-deficiency#:~:text=FALSE.,having%20too%20little%20vitamin%20D.

6 Alysha Herman, "The Link Between Tanning Beds and Cancer," Dr. Alysa Herman, accessed February 2, 2024, https://www.dralysaherman.com/articles/the-link-between-tanning-beds-and-skin-cancer/#:~:text=People%20who%20use%20tanning%20beds,risk%20of%20melanoma%20by%2020%25.

7 Skin Cancer Foundation, "5 Myths of Indoor Tanning, Busted!" January 26, 2024, https://www.skincancer.org/blog/5-myths-indoor-tanning-busted/.

8 American Academy of Dermatology, "10 Surprising Facts about Indoor Tanning," last updated April 26, 2023, https://www.aad.org/public/diseases/skin-cancer/surprising-facts-about-indoor-tanning.

9   Harvard T.H. Chan | School of Public Health, "Vitamin D," last reviewed March 2023, https://www.hsph.harvard.edu/nutritionsource/vitamin-d/#:~:text=The%20Institute%20of%20Medicine%20(IOM,to%204%2C000%20IU%20per%20day.

10   Merriam-Webster, s.v. "revitalize," accessed March 3, 2024, https://www.merriam-webster.com/dictionary/revitalize#:~:text=%3A%20to%20give%20new%20life%20or,t%C9%99%2Dl%C9%99%2D%CB%88z%C4%81%2Dsh%C9%99n.

Chapter 8

1   David B. Roosevelt, *Grandmere, A Personal History of Eleanor Roosevelt* (New York: Warner Books), 2002, frontispiece (without source).

2   Ken Ham, "How to Prevent Losing Another Generation," accessed January 29, 2024, https://answersingenesis.org/church/how-prevent-losing-another-generation/.

3   Cleo Wade, "everything that's happened," *Remember Love: Words for Tender Times* (New York: Harmony, 2023), Kindle.

4   Clay Jeter, dir., *Live to 100: Secrets of the Blue Zones*, Makemake (2023), Netflix, https://www.netflix.com/title/81214929.

5   Nancy J. Donovan and Dan Blazer, "Social Isolation and Loneliness in Older Adults: Review and Commentary of a National Academies Report," *The American Journal of Geriatric Psychiatry: Official Journal of the American Association for Geriatric Psychiatry* 28, no. 12 (2020): 1233–44. doi:10.1016/j.jagp.2020.08.005.

6   Christina Caron, "An Overlooked Cure for Loneliness," *The New York Times* | Well, December 21, 2021, https://www.nytimes.com/2021/12/21/well/mind/loneliness-volunteering.html.

7   Caron, "Loneliness," *New York Times.*

8   Caron, "Loneliness."

9   Caron, "Loneliness."

10   Susan Hunt, *Spiritual Mothering*, 2nd ed. (Wheaton, IL: Crossway Books, 1993), 45.

11   Gary Henry, "October 1: Uncluttering Our Lives," in *Diligently Seeking God: Daily Motivation to Seek God More Seriously* (Louisville, KY: WordPoints, 2003), Ebook, Henry_Diligently-Seeking-God_9781936357734.pdf.

12   Charles F. Stanley, *Every Day in His Presence: 365 Devotions* (Nashville: Thomas Nelson, 2014), Kindle.

13   Gary Henry, "June 13: Fruit-Bearing Discipleship," in *Diligently Seeking God*, Henry_Diligently-Seeking-God_9781936357734.pdf.

Chapter 9

1   Anne Graham Lotz, "Going Deeper in God's Word: A Bible Study from Anne Graham Lotz," September 11, 2017, https://www.billygraham.ca/stories/going-deeper-in-gods-word-a-bible-study-from-anne-graham-lotz/.

2   Graham Lotz, "God's Word."

3   Paula Williams, "From the Director—Trust but Verify," Special Services Corporation (SSC), May 24, 2012, https://www.flyssc.com/from-the-director-trust-but-verify/.

4   Jamie Waters, "Constant Craving: How Digital Media Turned Us All into Dopamine Addicts," August 22, 2021, https://www.theguardian.com/global/2021/aug/22/how-digital-media-turned-us-all-into-dopamine-addicts-and-what-we-can-do-to-break-the-cycle.

5   John Mark Comer, *The Ruthless Elimination of Hurry: How to Stay Emotionally Healthy and Spiritually Alive in the Chaos of the Modern World* (Colorado Springs: WaterBrook, 2019), Kindle.

6   Water Science School, "The Water in You: Water and the Human Body," USGS, May 19, 2022, https://www.usgs.gov/special-topics/water-science-school/science/water-you-water-and-human-body#:~:text=Up%20to%2060%25%20of%20the,bones%20are%20watery%3A%2031%25.

7   Corrie ten Boom, as quoted in Comer, *Ruthless Elimination of Hurry*, Kindle.

8   John Ortberg, *The Life You've Always Wanted: Spiritual Disciplines for Ordinary People* (Grand Rapids: Zondervan, 2009), Kindle.

9   Oswald Chambers, *The Oswald Chambers Devotional Reader: 52 Weekly Themes*, ed. Harry Verploegh (Nashville: Thomas Nelson, 1990), n.p.

Chapter 10

1   Teresa Nowakowski, "Merriam-Webster's 2023 Word of the Year Is 'Authentic,'" *Smithsonian Magazine*, November 29, 2023, https://www.smithsonianmag.com/smart-news/why-merriam-websters-2023-word-of-the-year-is-authentic-180983329/.

2   *Merriam-Webster*, s.v. "authentic," accessed February 9, 2024, https://www.merriam-webster.com/dictionary/authentic#:~:text=1,own%20personality%2C%20spirit%2C%20or%20character.

3   Nowakowski, "Authentic," *Smithsonian Magazine.*

4   Judy Garland, as quoted in Lou Kennedy, *Business Etiquette for the Nineties: Your Ticket to Career Success* (Charleston, SC: Palmetto Publishing, 1992), 8.

5   Missionaries of the World, "Robert Moffat," accessed January 30, 2024, https://www.missionariesoftheworld.org/2011/07/robert-moffat.html.

6   Jeff Donn, "America the Medicated," April 21, 2005, *Vox*, https://www.vox.com/2014/6/8/5786196/7-things-the-most-highlighted-kindle-passages-tell-us-about-american.

7   Joseph Stromberg, "Seven Things the Most Highlighted Kindle Passages Tell Us about American Readers," *Vox,* June 8, 2014, https://www.vox.com/2014/6/8/5786196/7-things-the-most-highlighted-kindle-passages-tell-us-about-american.

8   Mother Teresa, in "Faithful," ACTS International.

9   Henry, "Not What I Will (Aug. 1)," WordPoints, accessed January 30, 2024, https://wordpoints.com/not-what-will-august-1/.

10   Ralph Washington Sockman, as quoted in Henry, "Not What I Will (Aug. 1)," WordPoints.

11   *US Dictionary*, "You Go Girl: Definition, Meaning, and Origin," July 15, 2023, https://usdictionary.com/idioms/you-go-girl/.

12   Henry, "Window of Opportunity (July 3)," WordPoints, accessed January 31, 2024, https://wordpoints.com/window-opportunity-july-3/.

13   Kelsey Bjork, "10 Inspiring Viola Davis Quotes That Will Remind You of Your Worth," Inspire More, October 8, 2023, https://www.inspiremore.com/10-inspiring-viola-davis-quotes-that-will-remind-you-of-your-worth/.

14   Stanley, *Every Day,* Kindle.

BIBLIOGRAPHY

Allcott, Hunt, Luca Braghieri, Sarah Eichmeyer, and Matthew Gentzkow. "The Welfare Effects of Social Media." *American Economic Review* 110, no. 3 (March 1, 2020): 629–76. https://doi.org/10.1257/aer.20190658.

American Academy of Dermatology. "10 Surprising Facts about Indoor Tanning." Last updated April 26, 2023. https://www.aad.org/public/diseases/skin-cancer/surprising-facts-about-indoor-tanning.

Becker, Joshua. "Don't Just Declutter, De-own." In *Becoming Minimalist*. Podcast, 4:28. November 19, 2021. https://www.youtube.com/watch?v=-faHfZOdFiY.

Bjork, Kelsey. "10 Inspiring Viola Davis Quotes That Will Remind You of Your Worth." Inspire More. October 8, 2023. https://www.inspiremore.com/10-inspiring-viola-davis-quotes-that-will-remind-you-of-your-worth/.

Black, Christa. *God Loves Ugly: & love makes beautiful.* Reprint ed. Nashville: FaithWords, 2013. Kindle.

Brockman, Rob. "5 Biblical Principles for Social Media." The Gospel Coalition | Canada, September 27, 2021. https://ca.thegospelcoalition.org/article/5-biblical-principles-for-social-media/.

Buettner, Dan. *The Blue Zones Solution: Eating and Living Like the World's Healthiest People.* Washington, DC: National Geographic, 2015. Kindle.

Burket, Julia. "22 Facts about the Brain | World Brain Day - Dent Neurologic." Dentin Institute. July 22, 2019. https://www.dentinstitute.com/22-facts-about-the-brain-world -brain-day/#:~:text=About%2075%25%20of%20the%20 brain.

Caron, Christina. "An Overlooked Cure for Loneliness." *The New York Times* | Well. December 21, 2021. https://www .nytimes.com/2021/12/21/well/mind/loneliness -volunteering.html.

Cash, Amanda, producer. *The Oprah Winfrey Show*. Season 23, Episode 82. "What Can You Live Without Experiment (Pt. 2)." Aired March 2, 2009. https://www.youtube.com/ watch?v=Y7gk4Ur7-EE.

Centers for Disease Control and Prevention. "Adolescent and School Health | CDC." September 4, 2020. https://www .cdc.gov/healthyyouth/.

Chambers, Oswald. *The Oswald Chambers Devotional Reader: 52 Weekly Themes*, ed. Harry Verploegh, n.p. Nashville: Thomas Nelson, 1990.

Chartwell. "9 Lessons on Health and Longevity from the World's Blue Zones." 2023. https://chartwell.com/en /blog/2018/02/9-lessons-on-health-and-longevity-from -the-world%E2%80%99s-blue-zones.

Colbert, Don. *Deadly Emotions: Understanding the Mind-Body-Spirit Connection That Can Heal or Destroy You*. Nashville: Thomas Nelson, 2020. Kindle.

Comer, John Mark. *The Ruthless Elimination of Hurry: How to Stay Emotionally Healthy and Spiritually Alive in the Chaos of the Modern World.* Colorado Springs: WaterBrook, 2019. Kindle.

Donn, Jeff. "America the Medicated," *Vox.* April 21, 2005. https://www.vox.com/2014/6/8/5786196/7-things-the -most-highlighted-kindle-passages-tell-us-about-american.

Donovan, Nancy J, and Dan Blazer. "Social Isolation and Loneliness in Older Adults: Review and Commentary of a National Academies Report." *The American Journal of Geriatric Psychiatry: Official Journal of the American Association for Geriatric Psychiatry* 28, no. 12 (2020): 1233–44. doi:10.1016/j.jagp.2020.08.005.

Foco, Zonya. "How Many Servings of Fruit & Vegetables Do You Eat, Really? Zonya. Accessed February 8, 2024. https://zonya.com/articles/how-many-servings-fruits -vegetables-do-you-really-eat/.

Freeman, Emily. *The Next Right Thing: A Simple, Soulful Practice for Making Life Decisions.* Ada, MI: Revell, 2019. Kindle.

Games, Genesis. "The Impact of Social Media on Relationships." The Gottman Institute, February 10, 2022. https://www.gottman.com/blog/the-impact-of-social -media-on-relationships/.

Garland, Judy. In Kennedy, Lou. *Business Etiquette for the Nineties: Your Ticket to Career Success,* 8. Charleston, SC: Palmetto Publishing, 1992.

Graham Lotz, Anne. "Going Deeper in God's Word: A Summer Bible Study to Share." Billy Graham Evangelistic Association – UK. July 24, 2019. https://

billygraham.org.uk/p/going-deeper-in-gods-word-a
-summer-bible-study-to-share/.

Ham, Ken. "How to Prevent Losing Another Generation."
Accessed January 29, 2024. https://answersingenesis.org
/church/how-prevent-losing-another-generation/.

Harvard Health Publishing. Harvard Medical School. "Time
for More Vitamin D." September 1, 2008. https://www
.health.harvard.edu/staying-healthy/time-for-more
-vitamin-d.

Harvard T.H. Chan | School of Public Health. "Vitamin D."
Last reviewed March 2023. Harvard, https://www.hsph.
harvard.edu/nutritionsource/vitamin-d/#:~:text=The%20
Institute%20of%20Medicine%20(IOM,to%20
4%2C000%20IU%20per%20day.

Henry, Gary. *Diligently Seeking God: Daily Motivation to
Seek God More Seriously.* Louisville, KY: WordPoints,
2003. Ebook. Henry_Diligently-Seeking-
God_9781936357734.pdf. .

Herman, Alysha. "The Link Between Tanning Beds and
Cancer." Dr. Alysa Herman. Accessed January 30, 2024.
https://www.dralysaherman.com/articles/the-link-between
-tanning-beds-and-skin-cancer/#:~:text=People%20
who%20use%20tanning%20beds,risk%20of%20
melanoma%20by%2020%25.

Hippocrates, *The Aphorisms of Hippocrates.* New York: Collins,
1817, n.p.

Hunt, Susan. *Spiritual Mothering.* 2nd ed., 45. Wheaton, IL:
Crossway Books, 1993.

Jeter, Clay, dir. *Live to 100: Secrets of the Blue Zones.* Makemake (2023). Netflix. https://www.netflix.com/title/81214929.

Johns Hopkins Medicine. "Sunscreen and Your Morning Routine." | Health. Accessed January 29, 2024. https://www.hopkinsmedicine.org/health/wellness-and-prevention/sunscreen-and-your-morning-routine.

Kloss, Kelsey. "139 Nutrition Statistics You Need to Know." Livestrong. Updated December 22, 2023. https://www.livestrong.com/article/13731066-nutrition-statistics/.

Lamott, Anne. (@AnneLamottQuote). "'No' is a complete sentence. It's given me this tremendous sense of power. I'm a little bit drunk on it." Twitter (now X). October 18, 2017, 8:27 a.m. https://twitter.com/AnneLamottQuote/status/920657616707182592?lang=en.

Lewis, C. S. *Mere Christianity,* 87–88. New York: Touchstone, 1996.

Mayo Clinic. "Chronic Stress Puts Your Health at Risk." Mayo Foundation for Medical Education and Research. July 8, 2021. https://www.mayoclinic.org/healthy-lifestyle/stress-management/in-depth/stress/art-20046037.

Mehrabian, Albert. *Silent Messages,* 76–77. Belmont, CA: Wadsworth, 1972.

Mikel, Betsy. "1 Simple Way to Help Kids Perform Better at School (It Works for Adults, Too). *Inc.* March 23, 2017. https://www.inc.com/betsy-mikel/science-says-kids-learn-better-when-their-teachers-do-this.html#:~:text=Moving%20more%20helps%20make%20you,is%20great%20for%20your%20brain.

Mikhail, Alexa. "Loneliness Is a Public Health Crisis, Comparable to Smoking up to 15 Cigarettes a Day." *Fortune* | Well. June 15, 2023. https://fortune.com/well/2023/06/15/loneliness-comparable-to-smoking-up-to-15-cigarettes-a-day/.

Miller, Daniel P., Jane Waldfogel, and Wen-Jui Han. "Family Meals and Child Academic and Behavioral Outcomes." *Child Development* 83, no. 6 (August 7, 2012): 2104–20. https://doi.org/10.1111/j.1467-8624.2012.01825.x.

Missionaries of the World. "Robert Moffat." Accessed January 30, 2024. https://www.missionariesoftheworld.org/2011/07/robert-moffat.html.

Mother Teresa. In Richard Innis and Crystal B. "Called to Be Faithful." ACTS International. Accessed February 8, 2024. https://www.actsweb.org/articles/article.php?i=2597&d=2&c=2.

National Academies. "Sunscreen Does Not Cause Vitamin D Deficiency." March 31, 2019. https://www.nationalacademies.org/based-on-science/sunscreen-does-not-cause-vitamin-d-deficiency#:~:text=FALSE.,having%20too%20little%20vitamin%20D.

National Institutes of Health. "Vitamin D Fact Sheet for Professionals." Updated September 18, 2023. https://ods.od.nih.gov/factsheets/VitaminD-HealthProfessional/.

Nelson, Patrick. "We Touch Our Phones 2,617 Times a Day." Networkworld. July 7, 2016. https://www.networkworld.com/article/953059/we-touch-our-phones-2617-times-a-day-says-study.html.

Nowakowski, Teresa. "Merriam-Webster's 2023 Word of the Year Is 'Authentic.'" *Smithsonian Magazine*. November 29, 2023. https://www.smithsonianmag.com/smart-news /why-merriam-websters-2023-word-of-the-year-is -authentic-180983329/.

Office of Disease Prevention and Health Promotion. "Current Guidelines | Health.gov." August 24, 2021. https://health .gov/our-work/nutrition-physical-activity/physical-activity -guidelines/current-guidelines.

Ortberg, John. *The Life You've Always Wanted: Spiritual Disciplines for Ordinary People.* Grand Rapids: Zondervan, 2009. Kindle.

Piercy, Katrina L., Richard P. Troiano, Rachel M. Ballard, Susan A. Carlson, Janet E. Fulton, Deborah A. Galuska, Stephanie M. George, and Richard D. Olson. "The Physical Activity Guidelines for Americans." *JAMA* 320, no. 19 (November 20, 2018): 2020. https://doi .org/10.1001/jama.2018.14854.

Rabin, Roni Caryn. "What Foods Are Banned in Europe but Not Banned in the U.S.?" *The New York Times* | Well | Eat. December 28, 2018. https://www.nytimes. com/2018/12/28/well/eat/food-additives-banned-europe -united-states.html.

Regis College. "Does Social Media Create Isolation?" Regis College Online. December 23, 2019. https://online .regiscollege.edu/blog/does-social-media-create-isolation/.

Robinson, Patricia J. and Jeffrey T Reiter. *Behavioral Consultation and Primary Care: A Guide to Integrating Services.* Cham, Switzerland: Springer, 2016. Kindle.

Roosevelt, David B. *Grandmere, A Personal History of Eleanor Roosevelt.* New York: Warner Books, 2002. Frontispiece (without source).

Schrager, Sarina. "Integrating Behavioral Health into Primary Care." *Farm Practice Management* 28, no. 3 (June 1, 2021):3–4.

Shepherd, Sheri Rose. *His Princess Every Day Devotional.* Washington, DC: Salem Books, 2019. Kindle.

Skin Cancer Foundation. "5 Myths of Indoor Tanning, Busted!" January 26, 2024. https://www.skincancer.org/blog /5-myths-indoor-tanning-busted/.

Skin Cancer Foundation. "Skin Cancer Facts & Statistics: What You Need to Know." Updated February 2024. https://www.skincancer.org/skin-cancer-information /skin-cancer-facts/#:~:text=About%2090%20percent%20 of%20nonmelanoma,UV)%20radiation%20from%20 the%20sun.&text=Basal%20cell%20carcinoma%20 (BCC)%20is,in%20the%20U.S.%20each%20year.

Sockman, Ralph Washington. In Gary Henry, "Not What I Will (August 1)." WordPoints. Accessed January 30, 2024. https://wordpoints.com/not-what-will-august-1/.

Solon, Olivia. "Ex-Facebook President Sean Parker: Site Made to Exploit Human 'Vulnerability.'" *The Guardian.* November 9, 2017. https://www.theguardian.com /technology/2017/nov/09/facebook-sean-parker- vulnerability-brain-psychology.

Spence, Jacq. "Nonverbal Communication: How Body Language & Nonverbal Cues Are Key." Lifesize. February

18, 2020. https://www.lifesize.com/blog/speaking
-without-words/.

Stanley, Charles F. *Every Day in His Presence: 365 Devotions.*
Nashville: Thomas Nelson, 2014. Kindle.

Stromberg, Joseph. "Seven Things the Most Highlighted
Kindle Passages Tell Us about American Readers." *Vox.*
June 8, 2014. https://www.vox.com/2014/6/8/5786196
/7-things-the-most-highlighted-kindle-passages-tell-us-
about-american.

US Dictionary. "You Go Girl: Definition, Meaning, and
Origin." July 15, 2023. https://usdictionary.com/idioms
/you-go-girl/.

Wade, Cleo. "everything that's happened." *Remember Love:
Words for Tender Times.* New York: Harmony, 2023. Kindle.

Water Science School. "The Water in You: Water and the
Human Body." USGS. May 19, 2022. https://www.usgs
.gov/special-topics/water-science-school/science
/water-you-water-and-human-body#:~:text=Up%20to%20
60%25%20of%20the,bones%20are%20watery%3A%20
31%25.

Waters, Jamie. "Constant Craving: How Digital Media Turned
Us All into Dopamine Addicts." *The Guardian.* August 22,
2021. https://www.theguardian.com/global/2021/aug/22
/how-digital-media-turned-us-all-into-dopamine-addicts
-and-what-we-can-do-to-break-the-cycle.

Williams, Paula. In "From the Director—Trust but Verify."
Special Services Corporation (SSC). May 24, 2012. https://
www.flyssc.com/from-the-director-trust-but-verify/.

www.ingramcontent.com/pod-product-compliance
Lightning Source LLC
Chambersburg PA
CBHW020850090426
42736CB00008B/316